The 20-Minute
TRAVEL WORKOUT™

by
André Meintjes, M.P.T.,C.F.E., Ph.D.

Easy ways to stay active,
eat right and increase your
energy while traveling

No Equipment!
No resistance bands!
No gym!

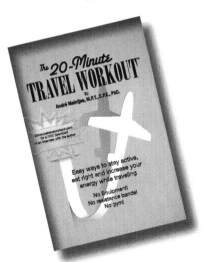

The 20-Minute Travel Workout™

TCH PRESS ✚

Meintjes, André M.P.T., C.F.E., Ph.D.
Book Design: Patty Atcheson Melton

1. Health 2. Exercise

Notice, the author of this book and accompanying programs used his best efforts to prepare this publication. The author and publisher make no representation or warranties with respect to the accuracy, applicability and completeness of the contents of this book. The author disclaims any warranties (express or implied), as to the merchantability, or fitness of the text for any particular purpose. The author and publisher shall in no event be held liable for any loss or other damages. Any person undergoing exercise regimens in efforts to improve or to maintain optimal health should first visit a licensed, qualified health care professional in order to first ensure whether he/she is healthy enough for exercise. Only such professionals are qualified to make a medical diagnosis and/or to prescribe medications or treatment regimens.

ISBN:978-0-9913758-0-6

Testimonials

As someone who leads a busy life because of work constraints and frequently travels, I was so excited to find a workout that was so compact and so efficient in just 20 minutes. The 20-Minute Travel Workout™ has it all! André has developed comprehensive whole body exercise routines that will take you to another level of fitness and productivity. I have even been recommending this to some of my patients who have been looking for something quick and efficient. If you are a person with limited time, loves to stay in shape, and spends more time in hotel rooms than your own, then this book and program is definitely for you.

Leigh R. Anderson, M.D.
Pulmonary and Critical Care Fellow
Board Certified Internal Medicine
University of Nebraska Medical Center

I have experienced the routines André designs first hand at the gym. Each routine is comprehensive in that it targets the whole body in a challenging combination of flexibility, strengthening and aerobic exercises. While traveling on business I am able to use these routines to stick to my fitness regimen. I'd recommend you take The 20-Minute Travel Workout™ with you on your business trips. Short, sweet, and effective.

Darryl Bader
Chief Operating Officer
ITS logistics
Sparks, Nevada

The 20-Minute Travel Workout™ is a jewel for anyone who travels or is just super busy and struggles to practice a regular fitness program. The routine includes flexibility, mobility, cardiovascular and strengthening components and is versatile enough for any fitness level. With this book, anyone can benefit from André's professional experience, education, and passion for a healthy and active lifestyle. You can maintain fitness and feel so much better while "on the road". I enthusiastically recommend The 20-Minute Travel Workout™.

Cathy Rich
Professional Sales Representative
Sacramento, California

Contents

Dedication

To my parents, Joan and Francois, and my brilliant sisters, Julia, Louise and Helen—I am blessed to have you as my family.

Acknowledgements

To all those who influenced my wonderfully fun childhood - you impacted my desire to pursue an active lifestyle from which the concept of this book originated.

Professor Duncan Mitchell, you are the brilliant mind who got me on track in physiology class and directly influenced me in my career choice - a magical teacher.

To my sons, Ian and Tate, you are a driving force for me. Thank you for being such fun young men to be around. I love being your Dad. Go easy on the old man when we are mountain biking!

To my wife, Coral - you are a patient, kind and beautiful soul. I could not have gotten this book written while running my clinical practice without you being supportive. Ian, Tate and I are so lucky to have your love and support.

To our model, my son Ian, thank you for going to the gym with me at 5 a.m. in the morning. He accepted a modeling fee of the Adidas outfit he modeled in!

Sierra Davies and Trevor DeRuise of Blü World Inspired, you took some great photographs and developed an awesome web site. Talent!

Finally, to all who travel – there is so much to experience in our world outside of our own little bubbles. I salute you for being out there doing your business deals, seeing how other cultures thrive, spending time with faraway family and friends. Enjoy your life's experiences!

Preface
Congratulations!

*Y*ou've Found a Unique System Designed to Easily Put You on Track for Improvements in Your Health and to Increase Your Efficiency.

The 20-Minute Travel Workout™ concept was born from multiple requests by fellow travelers who had difficulty maintaining their vitality and health while on the road. They felt pressured for time—engulfed in long periods of sitting motionless on planes, plus high-stress business schedules, often while being wined and dined. Yearning to stop being bogged down and to escape the sluggishness generated by cumbersome travel regimens, these people asked me for the easiest, quickest ways to become energized. Such requests impressed me as reasonable. After all, business travelers need to be mentally and physically sharp for peak performance in multiple business meetings. Yet travel routes make such objectives formidable for nearly all of them, unless using the tried-and-true strategies set forth in the pages that follow.

Indeed, I noticed the same challenges in my own travels, domestically and internationally. Just like most other business travelers, I recognized an urgent need for a quick, mapped-out method to keep my fitness and vitality high.

As an outpatient physical therapist for more than 17 years, I have been constructing short, comprehensive exercise routines for every one of my clients to complete at home. These routines supplement their in-clinic hands-on treatment. Developing the increasingly popular *20-Minute Travel Workout*™ evolved into a natural progression in my quest to improve the health of all travelers, rather than just executives and on-the-run sales professionals.

Determined to meet the specialized needs of these individuals, I used my extensive knowledge of the body and physical therapy in developing an overall workout regimen that entails "in-hotel programs" for travelers, preventing their bodies and minds from becoming stagnant while away from home. Business executives and other travelers now have the tools to improve their health, their decision-making abilities and vigor while on the road.

Thanks to *The 20-Minute Travel Workout*™ travelers can now focus on their specific business goals for each excursion. This unique, one-of-a-kind exercise regimen removes the need for you to decide how, when and where to exercise. *The 20-Minute Travel Workout*™ provides easy-to-follow, comprehensive exercise routines. All you have to do is pick a routine and do it!

We all know we must exercise for our health but we lack any knowledge of—or fail to understand—how this process should occur. Eager to simplify and to streamline the process into an effective universally accepted system, I provide you with the "how" and explain the "when." And as readers will soon discover, the "where" can become truly "anywhere" that you deem feasible. Simply complete a pre-constructed routine lasting 20 minutes.

This book is the first of a series from Take Charge Health, a public speaking and health consulting firm that I founded in April 2013. To meet steadily growing demand for additional advice, my follow-up books have or will feature:

- Newbie: A specialized publication packed with routines for new exercisers entering their first fitness programs at a gym.
- Health Maintenance: Look for my concise, "tell-it-like-it-is" report and strategy, an essential listing jammed with little-known but essential "insider" tactics necessary for consumers to keep themselves out of our super-expensive, budget-busting healthcare system. This critical and often overlooked process motivates consumers everywhere to take charge of their own well-being, becoming accountable for themselves while working to prevent health problems.
- Youngsters: Our "Take Charge Health for Kids Series" will teach your children, grandchildren or other young relatives how to benefit from healthy living. The beloved and adorable character "Baantjies the Baboon" and his friends help put youngsters on a pathway to healthy travels, enjoying lifestyles filled with excitement, health and productivity.
- Other publications: Bowing to public demand for more information on vital health-improvement processes, I'm also eager to provide additional advice in subsequent publications.

Take *The 20-Minute Travel Workout*™ wherever you go and have fun engaging in these beneficial routines. Feel free to email me your experiences at Takechargehealthspeaker@gmail.com. I would love to hear from you.

To your health and productivity,

André Meintjes

André Meintjes, M.P.T., C.F.E., Ph.D.
Founder and President: Take Charge Health

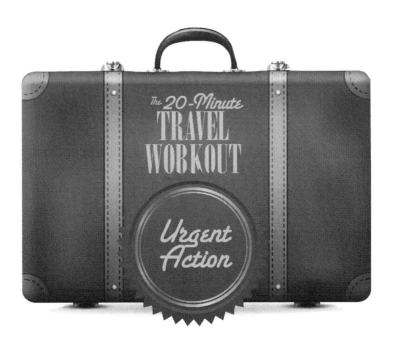

Chapter

1

Take Urgent Action Now!

*Y*ou need to walk for a whopping five hours and 48 minutes to work off a 1,613-calorie surplus generated on your flight to London!

If you're like the 99-percent majority of people, you lack the desire to spend virtually all of what little free time that you might have to eliminate these traveling blues. Now, you finally have this hot-selling book, *The 20-Minute Travel Workout*™ jam-packed with seven expertly designed routines of whole-body exercises to work off the unwanted stiffness and potential weight gain—while toning the body for maximum efficiency.

During a 10-hour flight from Chicago to London, you could easily consume a combined 2,303 calories from dinner, breakfast, a snack and beer or wine. The resulting danger to your health and mental well-being is primarily because during the same flight you expend only 690 calories just by sitting down for the flight. Thus, you have consumed a net surplus of 1,613 calories, and you would need to walk for hours to eliminate this excess.

When repeated over a period of months, years or even decades this process can result in obesity, while sharply boosting your chances for heart attack, stroke, accelerated aging and even cancer. Scientists and doctors warn that an excessively thick waistline virtually serves as a "proverbial oven for generating the deadliest cancer," drastically increasing your probability of getting many of the deadliest forms of this dreaded disease. Common cancers that oncologists often blame on excessive levels of body mass index or "BMI," primarily in the mid-section of the body, generate the disease in vital organs including the breasts, ovaries, testes, prostate, liver, lungs, kidneys and brain.

In 2007, the National Cancer Institute reported that obesity caused 34,000 men and 50,500 women to get the disease during that year. The institute went on to estimate that through 2030, an additional 500,000 people would suffer from obesity-related cancer. If each adult lost just 2.2 pounds, thus reducing their BMI by 1, the increase in obesity-related cancer would be prevented.

To help put everything here into perspective, you need to understand the fact that a pound of fat contains 3500 calories. Thus, on the Chicago-to-London flight the surplus you consume would result in 0.46 pounds of fat added to your body if not worked off, and that's in one flight. No wonder traveling challenges a healthy lifestyle.

Here is how I came up with these numbers. Dinner, a beer, a snack and then breakfast during the 10-hour flight to London all add up to 2,303 calories in and 690 calories out. While sitting on an airplane an average 170-pound male burns 69 calories per hour. Then the meals are placed in front of you with calorie counts ranging from 310 calories for a breakfast sandwich to 910 calories for 7 ounces of cheddar cheese pretzels or a 796-calorie treat pack and a 576-calorie snack box. The good old "peanut airline" seems to do better with its tiny 70-calorie peanut snacks or 50-calorie pretzels.

Cognizant and mindful of these critical dangers while

determined to easily avoid such pitfalls, take this book with you and enjoy my specialized, simple and fun exercise routines. In doing so, you'll quickly increase the probability of keeping those arteries open, and the heart pumping while preventing the waistline from expanding too much.

You will be glad you did.

After all, business travel increasingly hampers our ability to effectively manage time. Another challenge emerges from the fact that many of us often want to avoid exercise or neglect to follow healthy living standards when vacationing. Getaways can provide a much-needed break from the day-to-day norm of scripting all we do, while also attempting to escape the regular need to plan for food, exercise, family duties and work responsibilities. The multiple aspects of our lives rightly demand our attention. Yet challenges stemming from business travel and vacations can potentially endanger the vital time necessary to properly take care of ourselves and our families.

So, we must efficiently and effectively use each and every minute of each and every day during such excursions. Here is your guide to achieving this vital goal. You have bought this book because you made a decision to maintain a healthy lifestyle while traveling and you want to do it quickly and simply on your own time without sacrificing the reason for which you are on the road.

While traveling on business, we often feel pressured to maximize our time with the quickest, most direct, most cost-effective flight. You hit the ground with your cell phone to your ear organizing transport from the airport. Check in with the home office while in the cab on your way to the first meeting.

You have already become physically and mentally exhausted by the time the first meeting ends. Nonetheless, you rush to get a take-out dinner or a quick, unhealthy restaurant meal with a client.

Thanks partly to this rush-rush strategy, you have earned yourself the opportunity to benefit from a great workout, exercising efficiently at optimal levels—finishing just in time to clean up and prepare for your evening with your high-powered client. This additional meeting might result in big money for you! Yet in order to perform at peak efficiency both mentally and physically during that upcoming meeting, you must invigorate your mind and body. Up the energy! So, what should you do?

Exercise? Exercise?! Exercise!!

When vacationing many of us feel pressured to leave the hustle of home and work life behind and live each day on our own terms. Escape the rat race! No schedule! No mapping out every minute of every day in an effort to fit in the various aspects of your life. Normally you awaken early each morning to complete your one-hour exercise routine before heading to work, scrapping under relentless deadlines all day to maximize business profits, cart children to their multiple school and sports events, answer emails, texts and phone calls, spend time with your significant other and your wonderful youngsters and then read before crashing head-to-pillow—only to awaken in six hours to repeat this process. So, while vacationing, keep up your exercises with this short, efficient, fun *20-Minute Travel Workout*™—the whole family can join you!

How do you find 20-minutes in your day while traveling?

To complete a pre-designed, full-body workout that accomplishes multiple goals in a truly small block of time, you actually must schedule this vital exercise into your day. The best time for your first routine is immediately on arrival at your hotel room after the long journey during which you sat motionless for numerous hours. Get the muscles contracting, the ligaments and

18

tendons stretching and pulling, your legs weight-bearing, your heart pumping and those achy joints smiling because you make them do what they are meant to do ….. They are finally moving! Doing the first session immediately accomplishes more than just a physiological benefit. Exercise removes the traveling time cobwebs both physically and psychologically and sets the standard for the rest of your time on the road. Yes, you will now be on a schedule to maintain your optimal health through daily completion of *The 20-Minute Travel Workout*™.

Next, you should look at your traveling responsibilities and pick the best time for you to get in your 20 minutes. Are you most likely to accomplish *The 20-Minute Travel Workout*™ in the morning first thing and thereby invigorate your body, mind and soul for the rest of the day? Would you benefit more from completing these essential workouts after your busy day to calm the mind and body, thus preparing yourself for a good night's sleep? Will your sleep be negatively impacted if you exercise too close to bedtime, when a space of two to three hours before bedtime normally would suffice? There are thus only two factors to consider when scheduling your 20-minute session:

1. Which part of your day seems the most likely timeslot for you to get *The 20-Minute Travel Workout*™ done?

2. Do you have enough time between the intensive routine and when you go to bed so as to positively impact your sleep without disruptions?

Why *The "20-Minute" Travel Workout*™?

The 20-Minute Travel Workout™ workout time was designed with specific reasons in mind:

1. *The 20-Minute Travel Workout*™ is short enough to be accomplished quickly with maximum benefit. Time is of the essence when traveling. Factoring in exercise as well as clean-up time afterward, one can spend significantly more total time exercising than intended—negating the original idea behind the program, a time-conscious whole-body exercise regimen that benefits all physiological systems.

2. *The 20-Minute Travel Workout*™ is long enough to effectively target all parts of the body, through carefully selected stretches, strengthening exercises, balance activities, plyometric tasks as well as aerobic and anaerobic challenges with a warm up and cool down.

3. *The 20-Minute Travel Workout*™ specifically focuses on maintaining a degree of overall physical activity when traveling. It is not designed for the purpose of making you into a gladiator, an elite athlete or a muscle man or woman. This unique strategy keeps you active while on the road. There are other workouts, either shorter or longer. Typically, shorter programs target specific body regions such as abdominals. Longer programs may be designed to develop functional strength or a specific sporting need. They may focus on improving longer duration aerobic fitness or are part of a weight loss program. *The 20-Minute Travel Workout*™ activates, lubricates and invigorates.

What if I do
The 20-Minute Travel Workout™ consistently?

This depends on what level of fitness you are in, how you perform each routine and how frequently you define "consistently." I make a few assumptions here: you perform all exercises with the correct technique and at a suitable intensity for your fitness level. "Consistently" is at least three to four times per week, every other day, for four to eight weeks or longer, on an ongoing basis.

1. The Athlete: If in excellent physical shape thanks to an active lifestyle in athletic endeavors and whole-body training at a gym, *The 20-Minute Travel Workout*™ serves to maintain that level of fitness during your travels.

2. The Weekend Warrior: Consistently performing *The 20-Minute Travel Workout*™ will improve your fitness level, if already of average fitness with weekend participation in more rigorous activities. For such people, *The 20-Minute Travel Workout*™ emerges as beneficial because each routine challenges your body systems in a comprehensive way, thereby causing physiological adaptations that you fail to get from weekend warrior activities.

3. The Sedentary Workaholic: If sedentary, *The 20-Minute Travel Workout*™ undoubtedly will improve your health and fitness. You will benefit by performing these efficient, well-designed whole body routines, from flexibility to strength to aerobic and anaerobic capacity. Your health and wellness will undoubtedly improve.

How do I learn these routines?

Performing each repetition of each exercise in every routine with correct technique and intensity is vitally important. Correct technique limits your risk of injury when performing at the intended intensity. Every participant has a personal responsibility to take the time to learn the exercises well. In so doing you will maximize the benefits of the exercises, limit potential for injury and accomplish efficient use of *The 20-Minute Travel Workout*™ design.

Each exercise is described as follows: Starting Position, Movement, and Purpose. The "purpose" is identified as "WIIFM," an acronym designating "what's in it for me." Read the description of each exercise while looking at the photographs of the starting, middle- and end-positions. Then, when starting your initial *20-Minute Travel Workout*™, you should perform each exercise at low intensity with the express goal of learning to gradually perfect the technique.

Are you contracting the correct muscles to attain the ideal static position or to create the correct dynamic movement? Do you feel the stretches in the right places as described? Do you understand the purpose of each exercise? Spending time to perfect each routine optimizes your long-term benefits. Such concentration, careful attention to detail and learning will over time make each routine flow more efficiently.

The 20-Minute Travel Workout™ Philosophy

Each session is divided into four components: the warm-up; the whole body circuit; aerobic training; and recovery stretching.

Each component should take five minutes.

You should move at a controlled pace during the warm-up and the stretching while the whole-body circuit and aerobic routines should be done with great gusto and perfect technique. Your intensity during the session should remain as high as you can tolerate, producing a significant elevation of your heart rate, deeper and faster breathing as well as sweating. Rest minimally between exercises. This maximizes your time and yields the greatest benefit. Keep your heart rate elevated!

Each exercise is described in the pages that follow in this format:

1. Starting Position: Getting in the right starting position is important for completing the correct technique during the exercise.

2. Movement: Perfect technique every repetition of every exercise is vitally important for peak benefit and to minimize injury.

3. Images: Photographs of the exercises to help you visualize the starting position, a mid-movement position and/or an end position.

4. WIIFM: This "What's In It For Me" acronym describes each exercise's goal.

You have little time to get a challenging workout in so ... play hard, rejuvenate the body and mind from your travels and then create a successful business deal or focus on your family and friends!

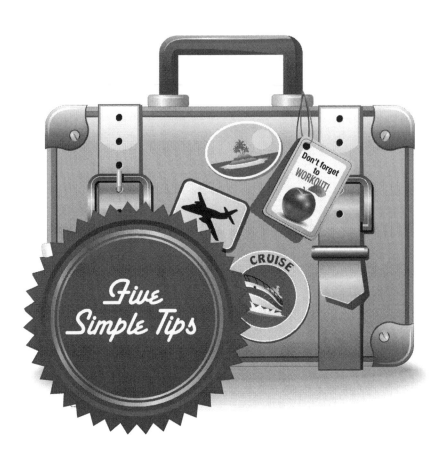

Chapter
2

Five Simple Tips For Eating Right While Traveling

$\mathcal{M}$ aking the right choices when eating while at home is not rocket science, and this decision-making process is no different when traveling. The need to attend vital dinner meetings, coupled with a lack of healthy restaurant foods emerge as the two biggest challenges that can influence your decision to stick to healthy eating while on the road. Your knowledge and desire to continue making healthy food choices should enable you to successfully choose the right foods when traveling.

So how do you combat these two challenges?

Access to healthy foods is limited while traveling due to various factors. Commercial airline passengers become captive to unhealthy, fatty and high-sugar airport and plane food as well as the outrageous cost. Rather than cave in to such temptations you should make healthier and cheaper choices by sticking to these five simple tips, the basics of eating right while traveling and while at home:

1. Portion size: Avoid pigging out!

2. Frequency: Eat five to six times daily, fully cognizant of Tip Number 1!

3. Monitor: Always review the content of each meal, particularly the ratio and type of fats, protein and carbohydrates.

4. Sufficient water consumption: Drinking water on the job is legal and safe!

5. Remain organized: It's easier than you think!

Bonus tip: Remain accountable to yourself—yes, it is your deal. Otherwise, you would not have bought this book!

Some airlines that provide meals also offer specific foods but only when requested beforehand, particularly on international flights. When possible you should seize such opportunities to continue your healthy eating. Airline security now permits taking certain foods of a certain size, usually up to 3.4 ounces, in your carry-on luggage through airport check points. Beforehand, check the airline for specifics. This simplifies the process of taking healthy snacks, while also enabling you to avoid unhealthy, poor-quality substitutes. When traveling in the USA, check with the Transportation Security Administration (TSA) Website at www.tsa. gov/traveler-information/traveling-food-or-gifts, or with similar organizations in other countries. According to the TSA, anything that has successfully passed through and been pre-screened at passenger security checkpoints at U.S. airports can be taken onto the traveler's designated plane. Success here hinges on your ability to organize beforehand, doing your homework in advance by checking the appropriate websites and/or calling the airlines. Once you've successfully completed this vital chore a first time, you will be set for future traveling experiences, remaining fully aware of exactly what you can and cannot take.

1. Portion size

Success here depends on using your hand as the measuring tool!

Breakfast, lunch and dinner should constitute separate portions of protein, vegetables and carbohydrates. Measure your individual portions by using the size of your hand. That is, a piece of chicken or red meat or fish should mirror the size of the palm of your hand in area and the thickness of a deck of cards. Separately, a portion of vegetables and a portion of carbohydrates such as baked potato or pasta should equal the size of your clenched fist. For example, an apple the size of your clenched fist is one portion or fresh carrots or broccoli, a cup of fat free Greek yoghurt or a protein bar.

2. Monitoring the content of each meal

Meal content refers to fats, proteins and carbohydrates. Within each of these there are relatively "good" foods such as olive or canola oil, seafood, whole wheat grains, and "bad" foods like chips, trans fat in cookies and almost any "feel good" food that can wreak havoc on your health including red meat, refined grains and sugar. Your goal is to eat from the good foods and avoid the unhealthy choices, so prevalent in airports, planes and anywhere there is a captive audience in need of a quick bite. Watch out because unhealthy foods can quickly sabotage your goal of maintaining a healthy lifestyle. Choose carefully using this simple knowledge. As I said, this is not rocket science.

3. Sufficient water consumption

Lots and lots!

Take your weight in pounds and divide it by two. The answer will give you an approximate number of ounces you should drink daily. For example, if you weigh 200 pounds you should drink 100 ounces of water or 10 to 12 eight-ounce glasses. By drinking these necessary amounts, you will spend time going to the restroom during the day, but maintaining optimal hydration levels within the body should always remain an essential objective!

Avoid confusing thirst with hunger which many of us do. Drink water whenever awaiting your next meal.

4. Eat five to six times daily

Your body and mind will need a relatively short period for adjusting to this new approach. Have a mid-morning and a mid-afternoon snack ready to munch. This should include fruits, veggies or whole grain breads, cereals or pasta, all consumed in the appropriate portion sizes! Always beware of excessive fat content.

5. Organize

In our busy lives we need to be efficient with our time and energy. So plan and schedule your food and snacks to coincide with your travel and meeting times. Since you travel frequently, have a supply of between-meal snacks at home that you can take on a moment's notice. Pack two per day, for mid-morning and mid-afternoon. Take a refillable water bottle, a cost-cutting measure, and drink, drink, drink. Think about this: the more you drink, the more you need to urinate. The more you need to pee the more you walk to the restroom. The more you walk to the restroom, the more exercise you get! If you wait too long and your situation becomes urgent, you will have to run to the restroom and that's more motion than walking! We can have fun talking about anything, can we not!?

Bonus tip: Remain accountable

Become "accountable," giving yourself the responsibility of striving to meet personal needs and goals. Anyone can be accountable for seven days consistently in matters that involve travel and business. How you exercise and eat during that time should be no different. You will be better off for it. You will feel better, and have more energy throughout the day, while maximizing your ability to perform at peak efficiency in your meetings and business duties. So get going and let me know how this works out for you. You can find my contact information at the end of this book.

Chapter
3

Exercise Routines

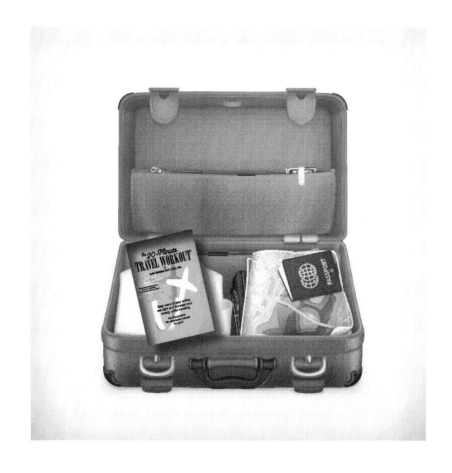

Routine 1

Quote for the Day

*I am what I am, I'm doing very well in my life,
and I'm thankful to God for that.*

-LL Cool J

Warm-up

1. Bend forward to touch your toes......X10
2. Hip crossovers......X10 left/ right
3. 90°-90° Stretch......X10 left/right
4. Gluteus bridge......3X10

Whole body circuit

1. Chair squats with overhead press......3X10
2. Push-up burpees......3X10
3. Superman......3X10
4. Partial sit-ups......3X10
5. Diagonal sit-ups......3X10

Aerobic

1. Ropeless rope jumping......1 minute
2. Mountain climbers......1 minute
3. Sprint on the spot (5 sec recovery).....3X20 sec
4. Jumping jacks......1 minute

Stretching

1. Hip flexor stretch......3X30 sec
2. Standing quad stretch......3X30 sec
3. 3-way butt-to-heel stretch......30 sec each
4. Press up with pelvic sag......X10

<u>Routine 2</u>

Quote for the Day

A good head and a good heart are always
a formidable combination.

-Nelson Mandela

Warm-up

1.   Bend forward to touch your toes......X10

2.   Hip crossovers......X10 left/right

3.   90°-90° Stretch......X10 left/right

4.   Gluteus bridge......3X10

Whole body circuit

1.   Static lunge......3X10 left/right

2.   Push-ups......3X10

3.   Lateral lunge......3X10 left/right

4.   Plank: front, left, right......3X20 sec each

5.   Floor touch squat-to-roof reaching......3X10

Aerobic

1.   Side-to-side jump......3X20 sec

2.   Sit-to-stand......1 minute

3.   Rotational jumping......3X20 sec

4.   Jumping jacks......1 minute

Stretching

1.   Hamstring stretch against the wall......30 sec left/ right

2.   Standing iliotibial band stretch and reach......30 sec left/ right

3.   Supine piriformis stretch......30 sec left/right

4.   Quadruped reach and lift......X10

Routine 3

Quote for the Day

It is health that is real wealth and not pieces of gold and silver.

-Mahatma Gandhi

Warm-up

1. Bend forward to touch your toes then extend......X10
2. Hip crossovers (90°-90°)......X10 left/right
3. 90°-90° Stretch with active rotation......X10 left/right
4. Single leg bridge......X10 left/right

Whole body circuit

1. Walking lunges......3X10 left/right
2. Chair dips......3X10
3. Mountain climbers with rotation......3X10
4. Overhead squat......3X10
5. Reverse plank......3X20 sec

Aerobic

1. Ropeless rope jumping......1 minute
2. Forward-backward arm leg swings......1 minute
3. Side-to-side skip......1 minute
4. Marching......1 minute

Stretching

1. Quad/hip flexor stretch......30 sec each leg
2. Iliotibial band stretch......30 sec each leg
3. Hamstring stretch......30 sec each leg
4. Standing calf stretch against wall......30 sec each leg

<u>Routine 4</u>

Quote for the Day
He who has health, has hope; and he who has hope,
has everything.

-Thomas Carlyle

Warm-up
1. Press-up......X10
2. Double knee to chest......X10
3. 90°-90° Stretch with active rotation......X10 each side
4. Hip crossover......X10 each side

Whole body circuit
1. Static lunges with alternate overhead press......3X10 each side
2. Push-up with clap......3X10
3. Burpees......3X10
4. Squat with diagonal weight press......3X10
5. Straight leg deadlift......3X10

Aerobic
1. Back-to-toes-to-back-to-toes......3X10
2. Alternate punch and kick......3X10
3. Marching with bicep curls......X10
4. Jumping jacks......X30

Stretching
1. Posterior cuff stretch......30 sec each side
2. Cat-camel stretch......3X10
3. Levator scapulae stretch......30 sec each side
4. Standing iliotibial band stretch and reach......30 sec each side

Routine 5

Quote for the Day

Happiness lies first of all in health.

-George William Curtis

Warm-up

1. Standing trunk rotation, shoulder level arms......3X10
2. Flexion in standing wide stance (Giraffe stretch)......3X10 left/ right
3. 90°-90° Stretch......X10 left/right
4. Gluteus bridge......3X10

Whole body circuit

1. Side squat with overhead press......3X10 left/right
2. Superman......3X10
3. Front plank......1 minute
4. Side plank left and right......1 minute
5. Chair overhead lift......3X10

Aerobic

1. Ropeless rope jumping......1 minute
2. Side-to-side shuffle......1 minute
3. Forward-backward shuffle......1 minute
4. Stomach-to-back up and downs......1 minute

Stretching

1. Hamstring stretch against the wall......1 minute left/right
2. Standing hip flexor stretch......2X30 sec left/right
3. Standing quadriceps stretch......2X30 sec left/right
4. Three-way mid-back stretch......30 sec each

Routine 6

Quote for the Day

The human body is the best picture of the human soul.

-Ludwig Wittgenstein

Warm-up

1. Flexion in standing......X10
2. Press up......X10
3. Hip crossover with trunk to follow......X10 left/right
4. Sumo squat......X10

Whole body circuit

1. Wall squats feet flat......1 minute
2. Half-burpee......3X10 left/right
3. Butt-to-bed touch single leg squat......30 sec left/right
4. Heels-on-bed straight leg butt lift......3X10
5. Single leg bridge......3X10 left/right

Aerobic

1. No-jump burpee......1 minute
2. Mountain climber......3X30 sec
3. Overhead wall touch......3X30 sec
4. Left-to-right weight shift with rope pull......1 minute

Stretching

1. Tricep stretch......2X30 sec left/right
2. Supine piriformis stretch......2X30 sec left/right
3. Standing upper thoracic stretch......2X30 sec
4. Prone gastroc-soleus stretch......1x10 left/right

Routine 7

Quote for the Day

Looking after my health today gives me a better hope for tomorrow.

-Anne Wilson Schaef

Warm-up

1. Flexion-extension-right-left side bending in standing...... X10 each direction
2. Upper thoracic to overhead to bicep stretch......X10
3. Knee-to-chest walk......X10 left/right
4. Walking quad stretch with heel raise......X10 left/right

Whole body circuit

1. Pushup with hip abduction......3X10
2. Reverse lunge to forward lunge......3X10 left/right
3. Stool scoot forward and backward......3X10 room length
4. Single leg bridge with arm raise......3X10 left/right
5. Chair dips......3X10

Aerobic

1. Jumping jacks......1 minute
2. Forward shuttle room run......1 minute
3. Lateral left-right room shuffle......1 minute
4. Squat with diagonal press......1 minute

Stretching

1. Tricep stretch......2X30 sec left/right
2. Supine piriformis stretch......2X30 sec left/right
3. Standing iliotibial band stretch and reach......2X30 sec left/right
4. Standing crossed leg hamstring stretch.....2X30 sec left/right

Chapter
4

The Exercises

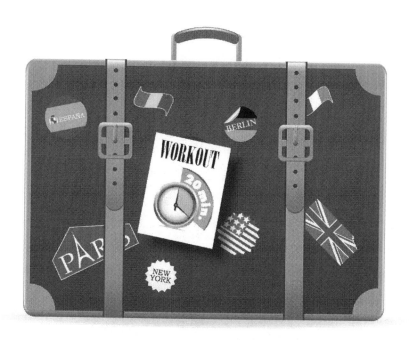

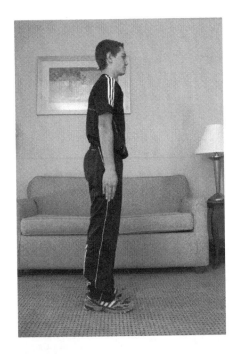

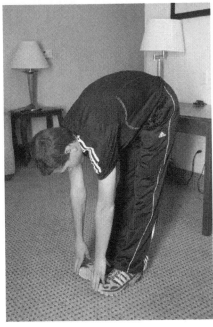

1. Bend forward to touch your toes

- Starting Position: Stand erect with your feet together and arms at your side.

- Movement: Bend forward starting from the top by flexing your neck to look down, then sequentially your shoulders (letting your arms dangle towards the floor), your mid-back then your low back. You should feel as if bending forward vertebrae-by-vertebrae from top to bottom. Bend as far forward as you can until feeling the stretch in the back of your thighs and possibly in your low back, particularly if you are tight there. Reverse the movement to return to the erect standing position. Keep your legs straight throughout the movement down and the return to the starting position.

- WIIFM: Improves lumbar and hamstring flexibility. Stretches the muscles and ligaments in your low back and hamstrings, the back of your thighs. Particularly beneficial after any prolonged sitting, such as after a long flight or meeting.

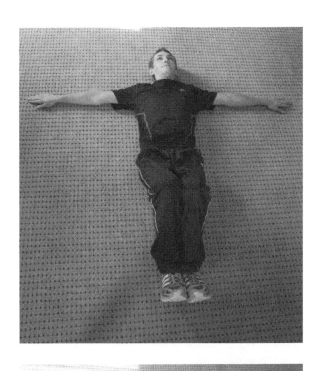

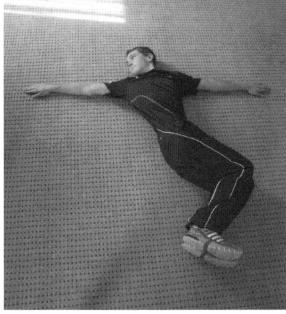

2. Hip crossovers

- Starting Position: Lie on your back on the floor with your knees bent about 90 degrees to 100 degrees. Keep your knees and feet together. Keep your heels on the ground and forefoot and toes pulled up toward your shins. Place your arms—palm down—on the floor, in line with your shoulders.

- Movement: Pull your belly button towards your spine and under your chest—make yourself skinny—thereby developing submaximal tension in your abdominal muscles. While keeping the abdomen tense, rotate your lower trunk to the left while reaching through the right hand and fingers. At end range, which is different for various people, relax your abdominal muscles allowing the weight of your legs to pull you into the stretch. Feel the stretch in your low back, abdominals and the right chest area. If you have been really tight, you may feel the stretch all the way down the right arm. Pause for two to three seconds, then tighten up the abdominal muscles again—make yourself skinny—and rotate your legs all the way to the right while reaching through the left hand and fingers. At end range, relax the abdominal muscles allowing the legs to pull you into the stretch. Repeat to the other side. Throughout the movement the feet and knees stay together and the heels on the ground with ankle dorsiflexed.

- WIIFM: This core warm up promotes mobility of the lumbar spine, stretches the core muscles and ligaments and creates low-intensity activation of the abdominal muscles.

43

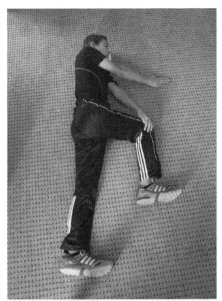

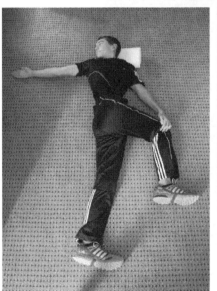
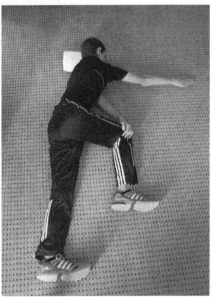

3. 90°-90° Stretch

- Starting Position: Lie on your left side with your left leg fully extended in line with your trunk. You can place a pillow or towel roll under your head. Bend your right hip and knee to 90 degrees and rest your knee on the floor. Place your left hand on your right knee, to keep your knee on the floor throughout the stretch. Place your extended right arm, palm down, out in front of you at shoulder level.

- Movement: Reach forward through the tips of your fingers of your right hand, thereby bringing the scapular forward and feeling a stretch between the shoulder blades. Maintain this reaching position while rotating your upper trunk and shoulders to the right, while also keeping the left knee on the floor. At end range, reach further into your right upper trunk rotation while exhaling. Relax into the stretch feeling this sensation in the mid to lower back. If your body has been really tight, the stretch might be felt along the inside aspect of the right arm all the way to the fingers. Hold the stretch for two to three seconds. Return to the starting position. Repeat on your left side.

- WIIFM: This core warm up promotes mobility of the lumbar and thoracic spine, stretches the lower quarter tissue of the core and creates low-intensity activation of the abdominal muscles.

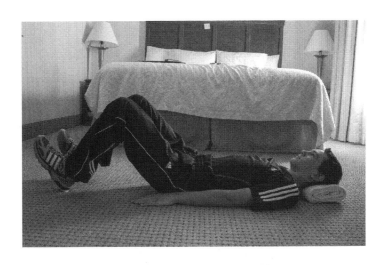

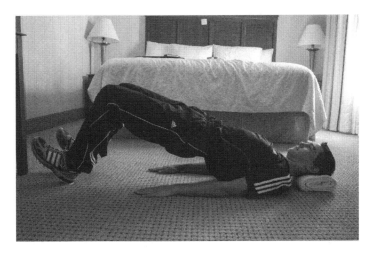

4. Gluteus bridge

- Starting Position: Lie on your back with your knees bent 90 degrees and your feet hip width apart. Place your arms on the floor, palm down, alongside your body. Dorsiflex your ankles so that only your heels are on the floor.

- Movement: Draw your belly button in to your spine and up under your ribs thus tightening your abdominals. Hold this contraction throughout each repetition of the exercise. Squeeze your buttocks together. Maintaining this glute squeeze, lift your hips off the floor pushing up through the front of your hips. You should feel your buttocks contracting together and pushing up through the central cleft and out through the front of your hips. Your fulcrum of movement is located through both shoulders—your trunk lifts up as a unit. Hold the lifted position long enough for you to ensure that you have a maximal buttock contraction and then return to the starting position. Without releasing the gluteus contraction, touch the floor with your buttocks and lift up again.

- WIIFM: Core muscle recruitment through isolated contractions of the buttocks and core musculature.

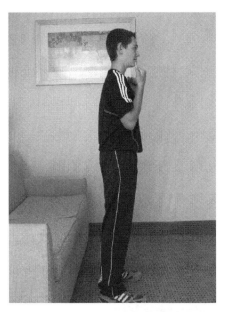
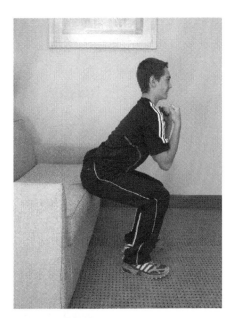
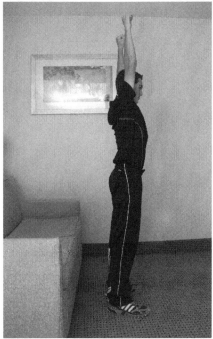

5. Chair squats with overhead press

- Starting Position: Stand with your feet a little wider than hip width apart, knees slightly bent, feet parallel to each other and with a stable chair that lacks wheels behind you. With arms at your side, bend your elbows such that your closed fists are in front of your shoulders, palms facing shoulders.

- Movement: Squat back and down as though sitting in the chair. Avoid sitting all the way down—only touch the seat of the chair with your buttocks. Your weight should be through your heels. Now, push through the heels of your feet, returning to the start position. As you ascend with your legs, push your arms directly overhead finishing with fully extended arms and palms facing forward. Repeat for the recommended repetitions.

- WIIFM: Whole-body strengthening through multi-muscle recruitment that involves the arms, upper and lower back, core, hips and legs.

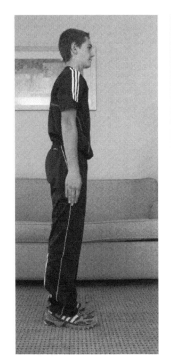
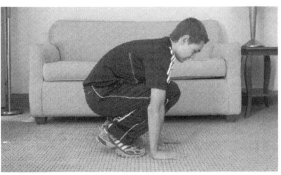
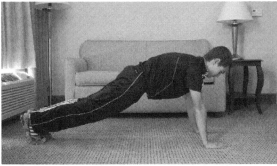
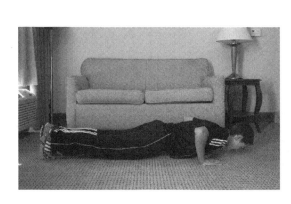
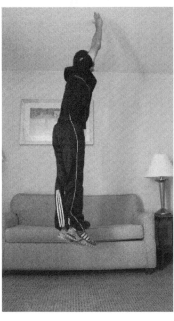

6. Push-up Burpees

- Starting Position: Stand with arms at your sides.

- Movement: Drop down into the full squat position with both hands on the floor just in front of your toes, elbows straight. Quickly kick your legs out backward so that you are at the top of the push-up position. Lower your chest to the floor and push back up completing a push-up. Immediately return your legs to the squat position and jump vertically as high as you can. As you land, repeat for the number of recommended repetitions.

- WIIFM: Rapid elevation of heart rate through multi muscle plyometric activation. A high-intensity exercise involving explosive movements.

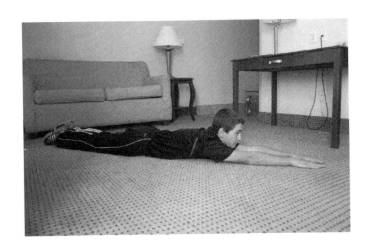

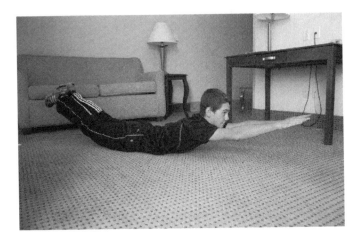

7. Superman

- Starting Position: Lie flat on your stomach with arms stretched out above your head and legs together.

- Movement: Lift upper body, arms, and legs. Keep hands and feet together. Feel a strong contraction in the buttocks, hamstrings and muscles on either side of your lumbar spine.

- WIIFM: Building strength and endurance of the paraspinal muscles up and down each side of the spine.

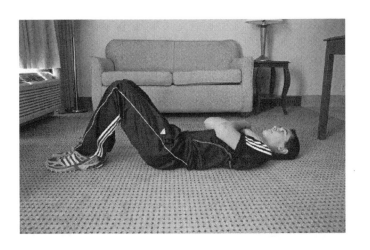

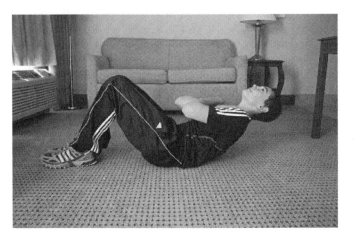

8. Partial sit-ups

- Starting Position: Lie on your back with your head resting on the floor, knees together bent to 90 degrees and your feet flat on the floor. Place your left hand on your right shoulder and your right hand on your left shoulder. Your forearms cross each other on your chest.

- Movement: Create submaximal abdominal wall tension by pulling your belly button in and up. While holding this contraction, raise your breast bone—sternum—vertically up so that your shoulder blades lift off the floor. The movement should feel as if being pulled up toward the ceiling by a cable attached to the breast bone.

- WIIFM: Strengthen abdominal muscles.

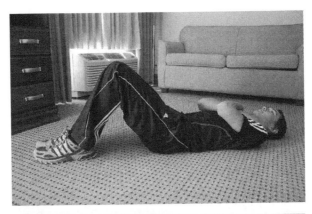

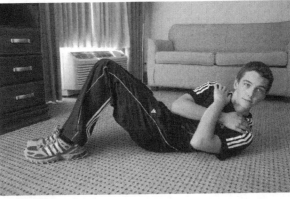

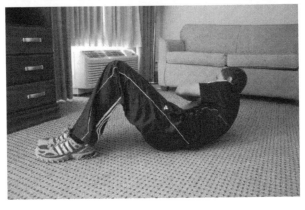

9. Diagonal sit-ups

- Starting Position: Begin in the exact position necessary for starting partial sit-ups (see #8 above).

- Movement: Create submaximal abdominal wall tension by pulling your belly button in and up. While holding this contraction, curl your right shoulder toward the left knee until the right shoulder blade comes off the floor. Return to the starting position. Now, curl your left shoulder toward the right knee until the left shoulder blade comes off the floor. Return to the starting position. Repeat cycle for the suggested repetitions.

- WIIFM: Strengthen abdominal muscles.

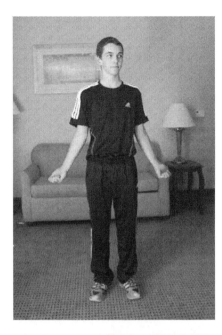

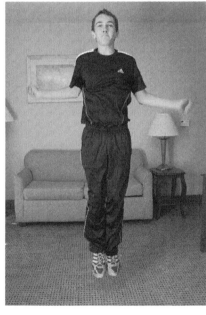

10. Ropeless rope jumping

- Starting Position: Stand with feet together and hands at your side as if holding onto a jump rope.

- Movement: Make arm movements and jump as if you were jumping rope. You can make any jump-rope patterns you prefer. With feet together while lifting knees high, jump from one leg to the other, left leg for ten jumps then right for ten. What you choose does not matter as long as the exercise elevates your heart rate.

- WIIFM: Aerobic conditioning through repetitive, submaximal activity.

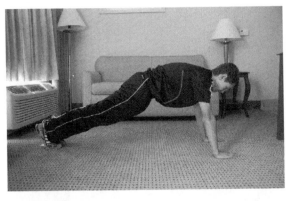

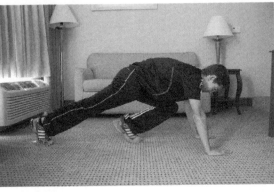

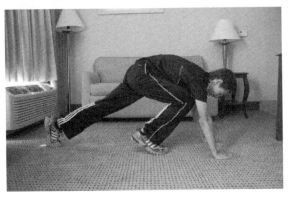

11. Mountain climbers

- Starting Position: Get in the push-up position with hands shoulder width apart and feet together, body in a straight line from ankles, through knees, hips, shoulders and ears. Keep elbows straight.

- Movement: Rapidly bring your left knee toward your chest, placing the ball of your left foot on the ground once the hip is maximally flexed. As you return your left leg to the starting position, bring the right knee towards your chest in a similar fashion to the left. Rapidly alternate left and right knees to chest for the required time or repetitions.

- WIIFM: Core control through shoulder and trunk stabilization during rapid leg movements. Aerobic conditioning when performed in sequence with other whole body exercises.

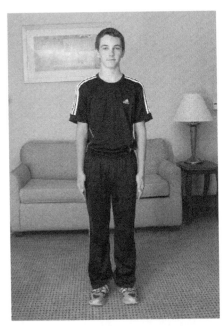

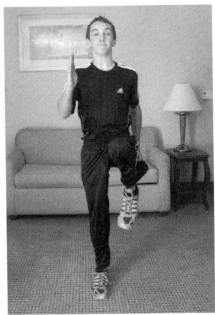

12. Sprint on the spot

- Starting Position: Stand with arms at your sides.

- Movement: Sprint on the spot using forceful pumping arm and leg movements as if sprinting as fast as you can for the required time.

- WIIFM: Develop anaerobic energy production through maximal intensity of short duration.

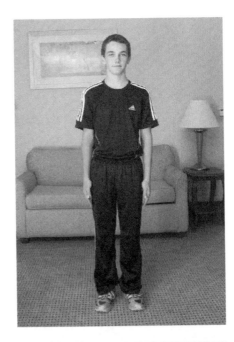

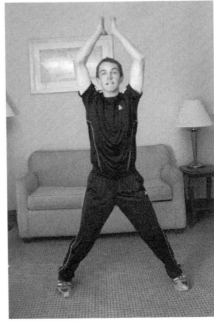

13. Jumping jacks

- Starting Position: Stand with your arms at your sides and palms facing in.

- Movement: Jump up spreading your legs apart and rapidly moving your arms overhead, keeping them straight. Clap your palms as they contact above your head and you land with both feet apart. Quickly switch directions and return to the starting position. Do required repetitions.

- WIIFM: Whole-body warm up through controlled use of multiple large muscle groups.

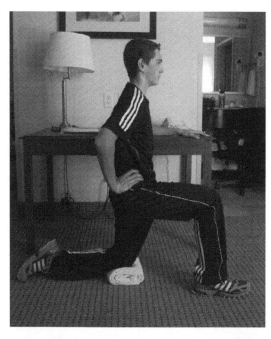

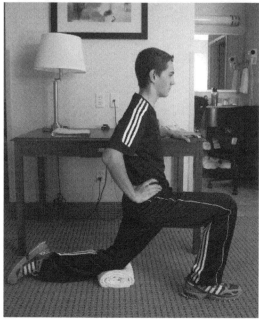

14. Hip flexor stretch

- Starting Position: Place a pillow on the floor. Kneel on the pillow with the left knee and place the right foot out ahead of you in a lunge position. Place your left hand on your left hip and balance with your right hand on the bed or table next to you.

- Movement: While keeping your torso vertical, tighten your left buttock pushing your left hip forward while shifting weight forward onto your right foot. The left hip is extended in this position. Feel a stretch in the left groin area. Repeat on the other side.

- WIIFM: Improves flexibility of hip flexors, especially beneficial after prolonged sitting.

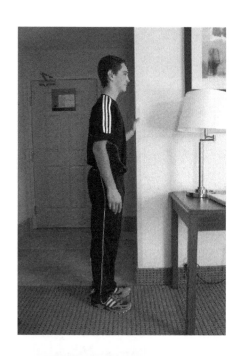

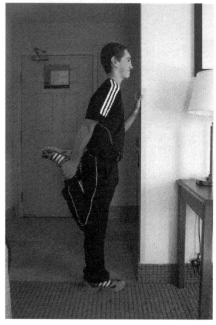

15. Standing quad stretch

- Starting Position: Stand on your right leg balancing by holding onto a door frame or corner in the room.

- Movement: Bend your left knee taking your heel towards your buttock. Grab the front of your ankle with your left hand and pull your heel to your buttock feeling a stretch down the front of your thigh. If you cannot reach your ankle with your hand you can do the same stretch lying on your stomach and pulling your heel to your buttock with a bed sheet or bath towel. Relax into the stretch for 30 seconds.

- WIIFM: Improve flexibility of quadriceps, beneficial after prolonged immobility.

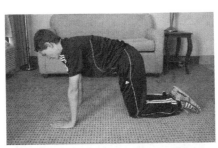

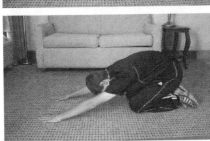

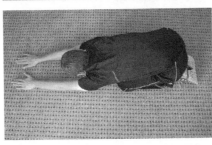

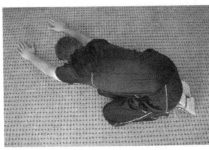

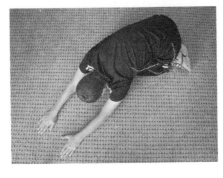

16. Three-way butt-to-heel stretch

- Starting Position: Assume the quadruped position with arms straight and hands a forearm's length in front of your head. Knees are vertically beneath the hips.

- Movement: Keeping your hands in place, gradually take your buttocks to your heels, tucking your head down between your arms so your forehead touches the floor when your buttocks touch your heels. Feel the stretch in your mid-back. To stretch your latissimus dorsi, lateral to the shoulder blades, perform the same movement with your hands placed to the right and then the left sides.

- WIIFM: Eases lower back and side stiffness following prolonged sitting or immobility.

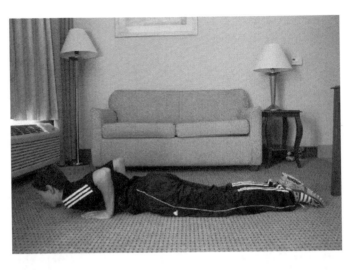

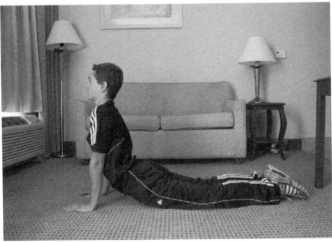

17. Press up with pelvic sag

- Starting Position: Lie on your belly with your hands under your shoulders in the push-up position.

- Movement: Relaxing your back, push up with your arms keeping your pelvis sagging and in contact with the floor. Your arms should become the only places in your body you should feel muscles contracting.

- *If you have low back pain and this makes it worse you should immediately discontinue this exercise.*

- WIIFM: Reduces lower back pain of disc origin and eases lumbar tightness due to prolonged flexed lumbar spine postures e.g. slouched sitting.

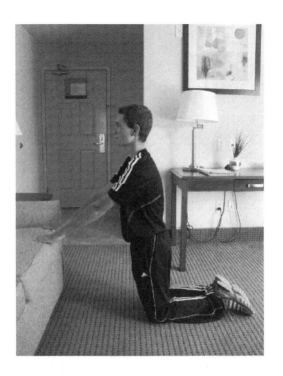

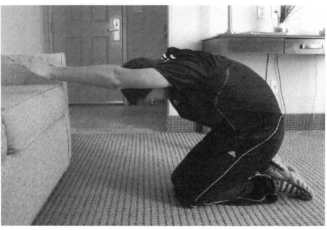

18. Quadruped reach and lift

- Starting Position: Kneel on the floor with both hands on a bed, chair or couch. Keep your body upright, fingers touching the bed, chair or couch surface. Maintain a torso-length distance between your knees and the furniture.

- Movement: Keeping your hands on the surface, gradually move your buttocks to your heels while keeping your elbows locked straight. As you descend, tuck your head between your arms, feeling as if you're falling between your shoulders. At the end range, attempt to lift your hands off the surface while keeping your body in the stretch position. You will most likely not lift them off the chair but your mid-back muscles will contract.

- WIIFM: Eases stiffness caused by prolonged sitting. This procedure corrects the problem by stretching the shoulders into full flexion, the latissimus dorsi muscles on either side of your trunk, and extending the lumbar spine. Lifting your hands off of the surface activates the mid-back postural musculature.

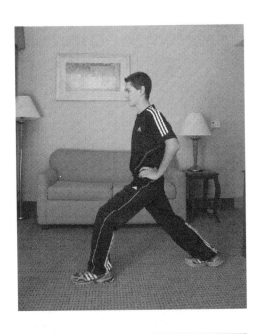

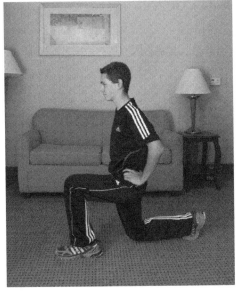

19. Static lunges

- Starting Position: Take a large step forward with your hands on your hips. The distance from the toe of your back foot to the heel of your front foot should be longer than the distance from your knee to the ground when standing upright. Your torso should remain erect and abdominal muscles tightened by pulling your belly button towards your spine and then under your ribs.

- Movement: Keeping torso erect and abdominals tight throughout the motion, lower your body by flexing the front and rear knees. Your front knee should bend to no more than 90 degrees, never passing the mid-foot. To think of "sitting back and down" can help maximize the effectiveness of this effort. You should feel your weight through the heel of your front foot, rather than the ball of your foot. Push back up to the starting position.

- WIIFM: Improves balance and strength through controlled activation of hip, trunk and thigh musculature with a narrow base of support.

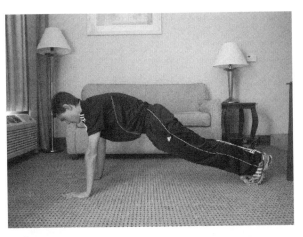

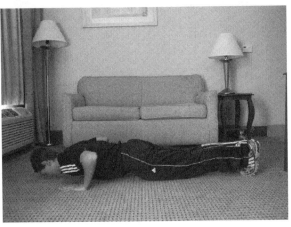

20. Push-ups

- Starting Position: Lie on your stomach with hands under your shoulders and elbows bent at your sides. Your legs should remain straight, with the balls of your feet on the ground. Tighten your abdominal muscles by pulling your belly button towards your spine and up under your ribs. Tighten your buttocks by squeezing them together.

- Movement: Keeping ears, shoulders, hips, knees and ankles in a straight line, push your body up by straightening the elbows to full extension in one smooth movement. Return to the starting position.

- WIIFM: Conditions core and strengthens chest and arm musculature.

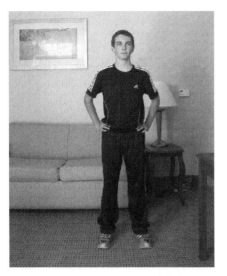
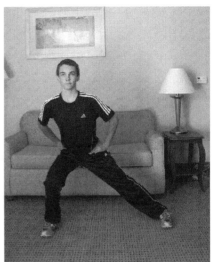
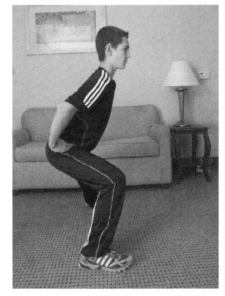

21. Lateral lunges

- Starting Position: Stand erect with feet hip-width apart and hands on your hips. Tighten your abdominal muscles by pulling your belly button toward your spine and up under your ribs.

- Movement: Take a large step, actually a lunge, to the right keeping toes of both feet pointing forward—feet parallel to each other. In a controlled descent, sit back and down as if you were touching your buttocks to the seat of a chair. The left-trailing leg should remain straight, with a stretch felt along the inside of your thigh. Staying down in the lunge position, bring the left leg in while keeping the right knee bent, thigh parallel to the floor. Step out to the right again and repeat. After doing the recommended repetitions to the right, repeat the movement on the left.

- WIIFM: Improves flexibility, balance and core strength through controlled activation of hip, thigh and trunk musculature.

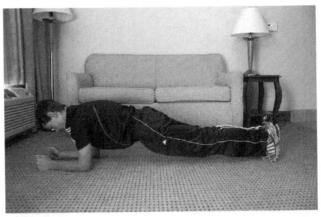

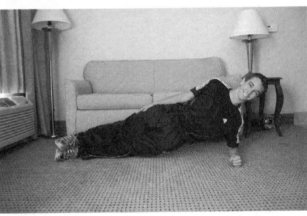

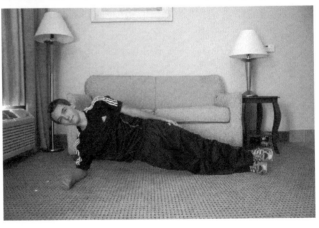

22. Plank: front, left, right

- Starting Position: Front: Lie on your stomach resting on your forearms with elbows under your shoulders.

- Left/Right: Lie on your side with your legs straight out and in line with your body, while resting on your elbow—the ear, shoulder, hip, knee, and ankle in a straight line, and upper resting arm palm down on your side. Keep the lower elbow immediately below your shoulder and your forearm pointing forward at 90 degrees to your body.

- Movement: Front: Tighten your abdominal muscles by pulling your belly button toward your spine and up under your ribs. Tighten your buttocks by squeezing them together. Keeping these muscles contracted, lift your body off the floor to rest on your forearms and the balls of your feet. Your shoulders become rounded by pushing through your elbows. Meantime, keep your ears, shoulders, hips, knees and ankles in a straight line. Hold for the recommended time and return to the starting position

- Left/Right: Tighten your abdominal muscles. Keeping these muscles contracted; lift your body off the floor to rest on your forearm and the outer edge of your foot. Your ears, shoulders, hips, knees and ankles form a straight line. Hold for the recommended time.

- WIIFM: Complete core stabilization exercises.

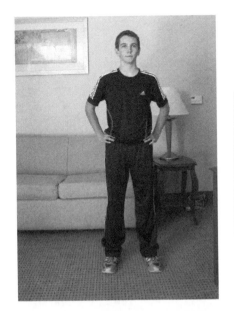

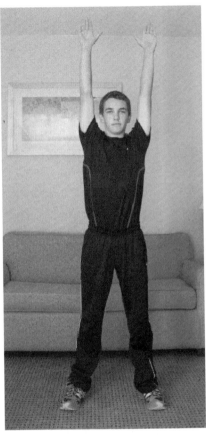

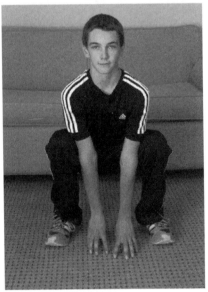

23. Floor touch squat-to-roof reaching

- Starting Position: Stand with feet just wider than hip width apart and arms at your sides.

- Movement: Squat down, essentially "sit back and down," and touch the floor between your feet with your hands. Your weight should be felt in the heels and not the balls of your feet if you "sit back and down" correctly. Your motion should feel as if sitting down into a chair. Explosively stand up erect pushing through the heels of your feet and extending your hips by contracting your buttocks. Do all this while reaching overhead with both arms as high as you can. Repeat for the recommended repetitions.

- WIIFM: Rapid elevation of heart rate through multi-muscle activation. This high-intensity exercise involves explosive movements to develop anaerobic energy production.

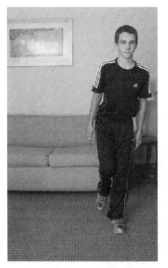
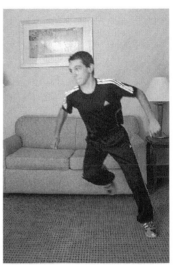

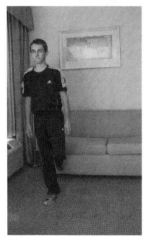
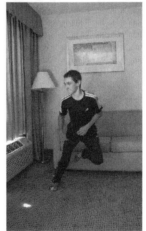
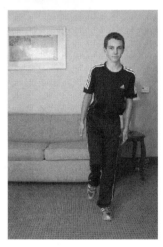

24. Side-to-side jump

- Starting Position: Stand on your left leg with arms at your sides.

- Movement: Concentrate on your goal of jumping to the right as far as possible, and stick the landing on the right leg. To do this, crouch down on your left leg and explode toward the right reaching as far as you can with your right leg. Use your arms to add momentum by drawing them backward as you crouch down on your left leg, forcefully extending them out to the right as you jump. Now, return to the starting position by jumping to the left. Repeat for the recommended repetitions. Start with a smaller distance until you have the correct technique and then increase how far you jump.

- WIIFM: Develops hip strength and proprioception for balance through explosive jumping and controlled landing.

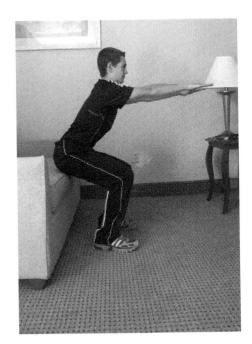

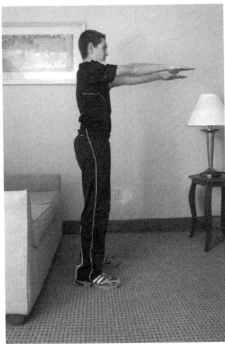

25. Sit-to-stand

- Starting Position: Sit on the front of the chair seat, feet flat on the ground. Beforehand, adjust this furniture's height so that your thighs become parallel to the floor and your knees are at 90 degrees. Your torso should become upright, the body's core braced by contracting your abdominal muscles. To accomplish this, pull your belly button in toward your spine and up under your ribs. Place your arms out in front of you at shoulder height with palms facing down.

- Movement: Stand tall while keeping the core of your body braced and arms out in front of you at shoulder level. Then, immediately return to touch the seat with your buttocks—sitting "back down," the weight through your heels rather than the ball of your foot. Actually, you must avoid fully sitting back down; just touch the seat with your buttocks. This maintains muscle activation throughout each repetition. Repeat the recommended repetitions.

- WIIFM: Strengthens legs, promotes balance and stabilizes trunk.

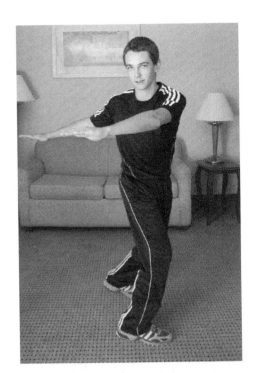

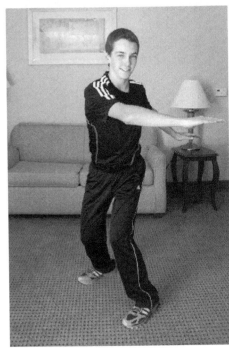

26. Rotational jumping

- Starting Position: Stand on the balls of your feet, with feet a little wider apart than hip width, and with elbows bent, arms approximately 45 degrees out to the side.

- Movement: Rapidly jump up twisting your feet to the left and your torso to the right and immediately upon landing do the same motion in the opposite direction. Continuously rotate as fast as possible to the left and right for the entire duration of the set. You should be breathless after each set.

- WIIFM: Establishes core and plyometric control through maximal intensity, short duration, explosive movement.

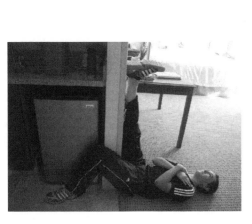

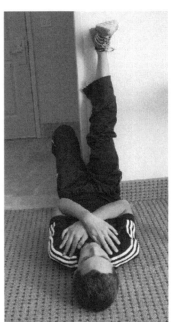

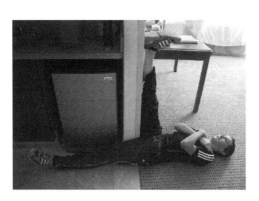

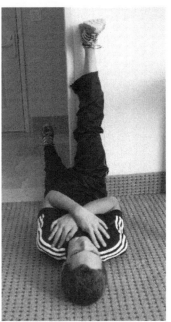

27. Hamstring stretch against the wall

- Starting Position: Lie on your back with the right leg through the doorway, knee bent, and foot flat on the floor. With the knee straight, position your left leg up against the wall to the left of the door frame. The left buttock needs to remain flush with the wall.

- Movement: Gradually lower your right leg until feeling a stretch in the back of the left thigh. Keep your left knee straight and flush against the wall. People with poor hamstring flexibility may be unable to straighten their right leg to the floor and/or initially be unable to get your left knee flush against the wall. Hold the stretch for the required duration. Repeat on the other side.

- WIIFM: Improves hamstring—posterior thigh—flexibility, especially helpful after prolonged sitting.

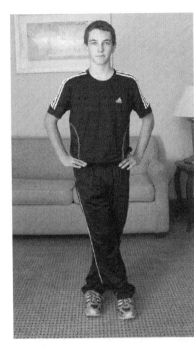

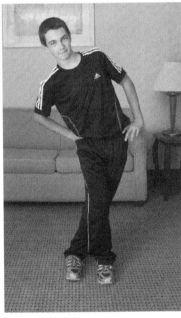

28. Standing iliotibial band stretch and reach

- Starting Position: While standing, cross your right leg in front of the left, keeping the left knee straight. Place your right hand on your right hip.

- Movement: While pushing your pelvis to the left with your right hand, bend to the right and reach overhead with your left arm stretching up and over to the right through your fingers. You should feel a stretch down the side of your torso and over your left hip down the side of your thigh. Hold for the recommended duration and return to the starting position. Repeat on the other side.

- WIIFM: Improve lateral thigh flexibility, also called the "iliotibial band."

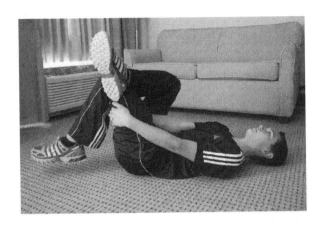

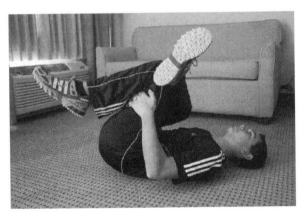

29. Supine piriformis stretch

- Starting Position: Lie on your back with your knees bent. Cross your right leg over your left, the right ankle across your left thigh above the knee—the Figure 4 position. Pass your right hand around the inside of your left thigh and your left hand around the outside to clasp fingers together around your thigh just below the left knee.

- Movement: Use your arms to pull your left thigh to your chest. In the process, relax your body until feeling a stretch in the right buttock. Hold for the recommended duration and repeat on the other side.

- WIIFM: Improve piriformis flexibility, especially helpful after prolonged sitting.

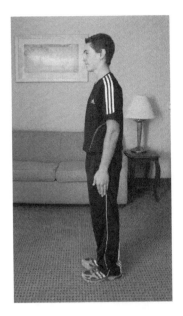

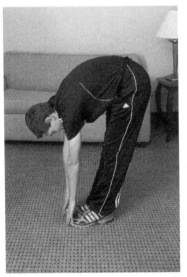

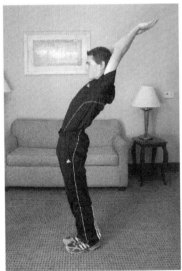

30. Bend forward to touch your toes then extend

- Starting Position: Stand erect with your feet together and arms at your side.

- Movement: Bend forward starting from the top by flexing your neck to look down, then sequentially your shoulders, mid-back and your low back. Let your arms dangle toward the floor. You should feel as if each vertebra is rolling down vertebrae-by-vertebrae, from top to bottom. Bend as far forward as you can until feeling a stretch in the back of your thighs and possibly in your low back. This will depend on whether your muscles have been tight there. Reverse the movement to return to the erect standing position. Now, place your hands on your hips and bend backwards. Keep your legs straight throughout the movement down and back, before returning to the start position. Repeat for the recommended repetitions.

- WIIFM: Improves lumbar spine motion and hamstring flexibility. Stretches the muscles and ligaments in your low back and hamstrings at the back of your thighs. Extending the lumbar spine stretches the front trunk or abdominal musculature of the body. This is particularly beneficial after any prolonged sitting, such as following a flight or a meeting.

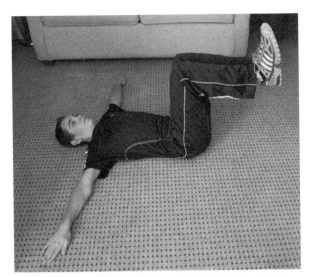

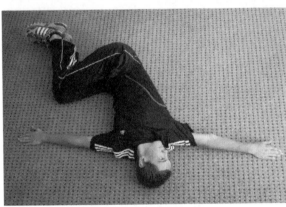

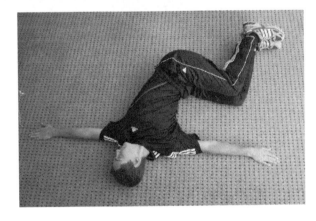

31. Hip crossovers (90°-90°)

- Starting Position: Lie on your back on the floor with your hips and knees bent 90 degrees. Point your thighs up vertically, keeping shins parallel to the floor with knees and feet together. Also keep your feet and toes flexed toward your shins. Place your arms palm down on the floor in line with your shoulders.

- Movement: Pull your belly button towards your spine and under your chest, essentially "making yourself skinny." This braces your core by developing tension in your abdominal muscles. While keeping abdominals tense, rotate your lower trunk to the left while reaching through the right hand and fingers. At end range, which is unique for each individual, relax your abdominal muscles. This allows the weight of your legs to pull you into the stretch. Feel the stretch in your low back, abdominals and the right chest area. If you lack flexibility, you may feel the stretch all the way down the right arm. Pause for two to three seconds, then tighten up the abdominal muscles again and rotate your legs all the way to the right while reaching through the left hand and fingers. At end range, relax the abdominal muscles allowing the legs to pull you into the stretch. Repeat on the other side. Throughout the movement the feet and knees stay together.

- WIIFM: This core warm up promotes mobility of the lumbar spine, stretches the core muscles and ligaments and creates low-intensity activation of the abdominal muscles. Advancement from hip crossovers.

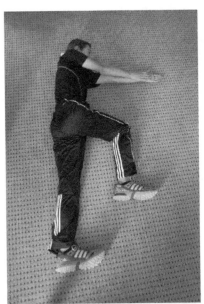

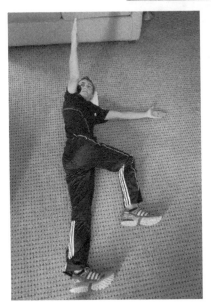

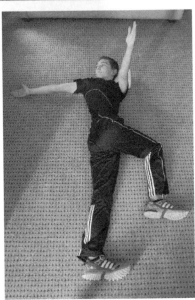

32. 90°-90° Stretch with active rotation

- Starting Position: Lie on your left side with your left leg fully extended in line with your trunk. Place a pillow or towel roll under your head. Bend your right hip and knee to 90 degrees and rest your knee on a rolled up towel about 8 inches in diameter. Your right foot rests on the floor in front of the left leg. Place your left arm on the floor in line with your shoulders, palm up and your right arm on top of the left.

- Movement: Keeping your right arm straight, raise your right arm up to point directly to the ceiling while pushing your right knee into the towel roll. This activates your abdominal muscles by actively rotating the lower torso to the left. As your right arm reaches the vertical position begin rotating your upper torso and your left arm in unison with the right arm. Keep pressure on the towel with your right knee throughout the motion. At end range with your right arm close to the floor behind you and your left arm pointing to the ceiling, reach through the fingers of each hand. This increases the core muscle activity in the opposite direction to that of the lower trunk rotation. Hold the contraction for two to three seconds. Return to the starting position. Repeat in the right side lying position.

- WIIFM: This core warm up and recruitment promotes mobility of the lumbar and thoracic spine, stretches the lower quarter tissue of the core and activates the abdominal muscles. This one feels really good!

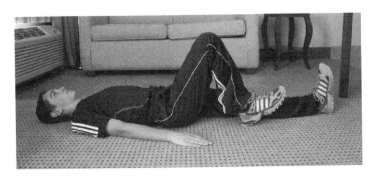

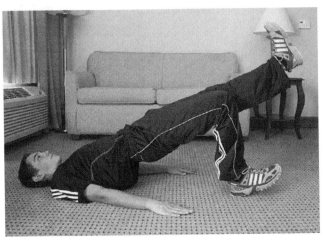

33. Single leg bridge

- Starting Position: Lie on your back with your right knee bent 90 degrees and your foot on the floor in line with your right hip. Dorsiflex your right ankle so that only your heel remains on the floor.

- Movement: Draw your belly button in to your spine and up under your ribs thus tightening your abdominals. Hold this contraction throughout the exercise. Squeeze your buttocks together. Maintaining this gluteus maximus squeeze, lift your hips off the floor pushing up through the front of your right hip and maintaining your pelvis level. You should feel your right buttock contracting more than the left and pushing up through the front of your right hip. Your trunk moves upward as a unit, the fulcrum of movement through both shoulders. You may notice that when performing this exercise the body fails to attain full hip extension, as experienced when both legs push up together during the regular gluteus bridge exercise. Hold the lifted position long enough for you to ensure that you have a maximal buttock contraction and then return to the starting position. Without releasing the gluteus contraction, touch the floor with your buttocks and lift up again. Repeat on the other side.

- WIIFM: Core muscle recruitment through unilateral isolated contractions of the buttocks and core musculature. Advancement from gluteus bridge exercise.

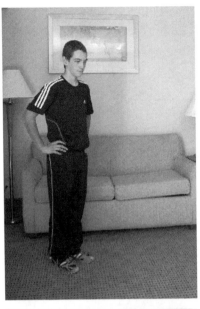 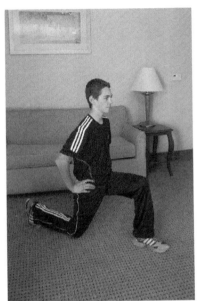

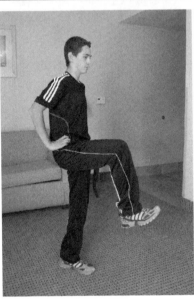 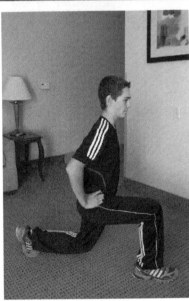

34. Walking lunges

- Starting Position: Stand erect with abdominals braced by pulling belly button towards your spine and under your ribs. Keep feet together and hands on your hips.

- Movement: Take a large step forward while keeping your hands on your hips and your torso erect. The distance from the toe of your back foot to the heel of your front foot should be larger than the distance from your knee to the ground when standing upright. Lower your body by flexing the front and rear knees. Your front knee should bend to no more than 90 degrees, never passing forward of the mid-foot. To do this, think of "sitting back and down." You should feel your weight through the heel of your front foot rather than the ball. Step through with the back leg while pushing up with the front leg into another lunge. Continue walking lunges for the recommended repetitions.

- WIIFM: Develops dynamic balance, core control and leg strength.

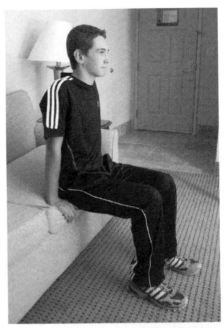

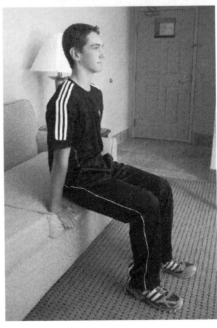

35. Chair dips

- Starting Position: Use a stable chair with arm rests and without wheels. If your room lacks such furniture then use your fists on the floor. Sit in the stable chair with your feet flat on the floor and knees bent at 90 degrees. Place your hands on each arm rest and straighten your elbows thereby lifting your buttocks off the seat of the chair. You torso should remain vertical below your shoulders.

- Movement: Lower your buttocks toward the seat by "sinking" between your shoulders, while maintaining elbows locked in full extension. Now, raise your buttocks away from the seat of the chair by pushing up vertically through your locked arms. Your torso should rise as your shoulders move down. Repeat for the recommended repetitions.

- WIIFM: Strengthens the triceps at the back of the upper arms, and the inferior trapezius muscles that stabilize the shoulder blades during arm use. Passively straightens—tractions—the lower back, relieving pressure in the spine, a problem often caused by prolonged sitting.

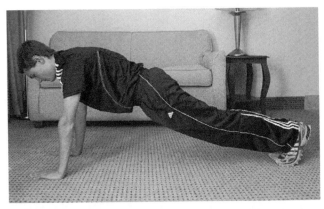

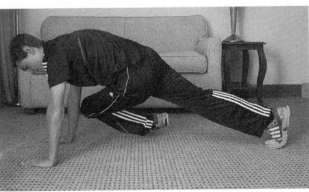

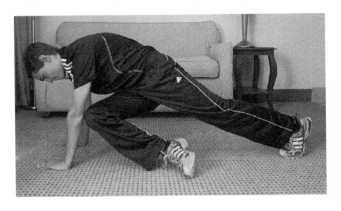

36. Mountain climbers with rotation

- Starting Position: Get in the push-up position with hands shoulder width apart, feet together and elbows straight. Keep your body in a straight line from ankles, through knees, hips, shoulders and ears.

- Movement: Bring your left knee toward your right elbow. Without placing your foot on the ground, return your left leg to the starting position. Bring the right knee toward your left elbow in a similar fashion to the left. Alternate left and right knees to opposite elbows for the required time or repetitions.

- WIIFM: Core control and flexibility through the trunk and shoulder during slow diagonal leg movements.

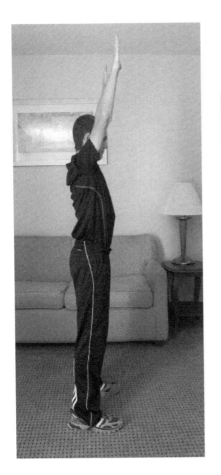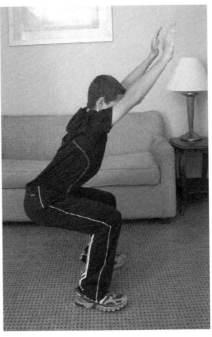

37. Overhead squat

- Starting Position: Stand with your feet a little wider than hip width apart, knees slightly bent, and feet parallel to each other. Keep your arms overhead while reaching through your fingers toward the ceiling. You should feel your entire body stretch upward.

- Movement: Maintain this erect posture, reaching up through your fingers above your head. Squat back and down as though sitting in a chair. You should feel your weight through the heels, rather than the balls of your feet. As your body descends, the knees never pass beyond the mid-foot. Squat down until your thighs become parallel to the floor. Now, return to the starting position, pushing through the heels. Complete the recommended repetitions.

- WIIFM: Whole-body strengthening and improving the flexibility of the thoracic spine—accomplished by overhead reaching, plus the working of a multi-muscle group consisting of the arms, upper and lower back, core, hips and legs.

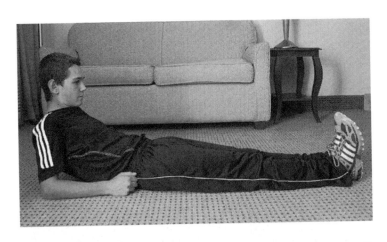

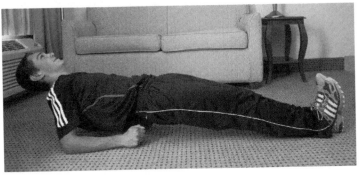

38. Reverse plank

- Starting Position: Lie on your back resting on your forearms with elbows under your shoulders. Keep your body relaxed on the floor as if you are looking out to sea while on a beach. Keep your legs and feet together.

- Movement: Brace your abdominal muscles by pulling your belly button toward your spine and up under your ribs. Squeeze your buttocks together and lift your body off the floor feeling the buttocks push up through the front of your hips. At the top of the movement you should rest on your forearms and heels, with shoulders pulled back and down as if sticking your chest out. Keep your ears, shoulders, hips, knees and ankles in a straight line. Hold for the recommended time and return to the starting position.

- WIIFM: Complete core stabilization exercise emphasizes back muscles, buttocks and hamstrings.

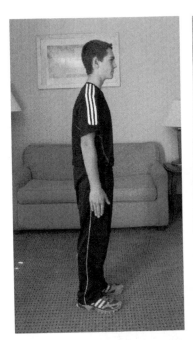
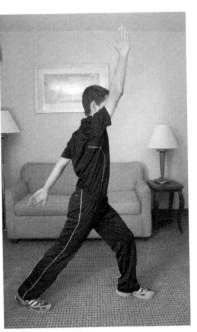
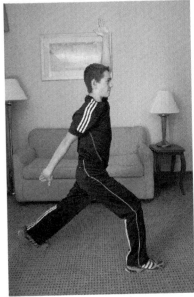

39. Forward-backward arm leg swings

- Starting Position: Stand with feet together and arms at your side, palms facing your thighs.

- Movement: Your arms and legs remain straight throughout this exercise. Rapidly swing your arms and legs forward and backward as if marching on the spot. Use full arm and leg range of motion. Continue for the recommended time.

- WIIFM: Aerobic conditioning through prolonged, repetitive, submaximal use of multiple large muscle groups.

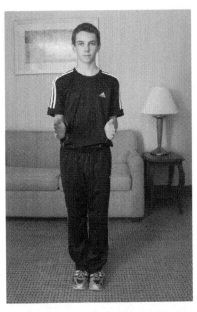

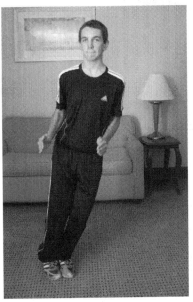

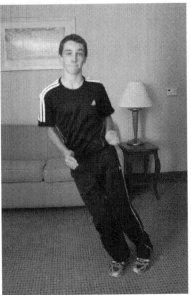

40. Side-to-side skip

- Starting Position: Stand with feet and knees together and arms at your sides, elbows bent at 90 degrees so forearms become parallel to the floor.

- Movement: Imagine a line immediately next to your right foot. Your goal is to skip across this line and back as fast as you can for the recommended time, landing and exploding of the balls of your feet. Keep your feet and knees together, similar to a skiing motion. The knees and hips should remain slightly bent to absorb shock, while extended forcefully to create the lateral movement.

- WIIFM: Develops leg strength and control of explosive movements through rapid, maximal speed activity.

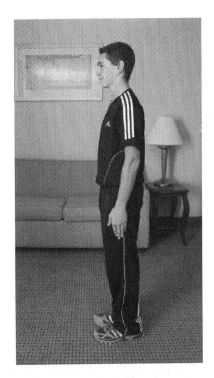

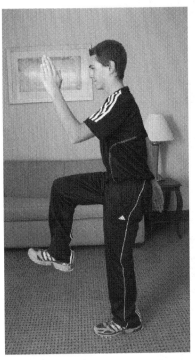 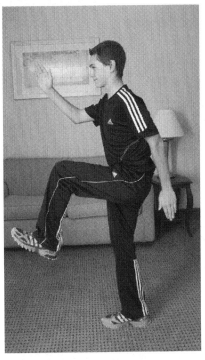

41. Marching

- Starting Position: Stand with feet together and arms at your side.

- Movement: Rapidly march on the spot lifting your thighs parallel to the floor while swinging your opposite arms up to shoulder height. Continue for the recommended time.

- WIIFM: Aerobic conditioning through prolonged, repetitive, submaximal use of multiple large muscle groups.

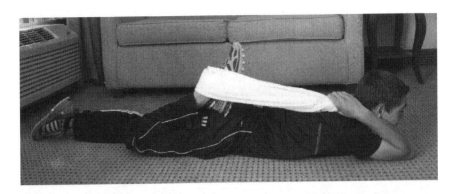

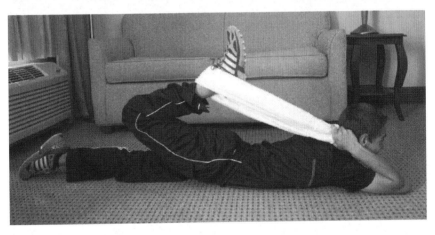

42. Quad/hip flexor stretch

- Starting Position: Lie prone with a bed sheet or bath towel around your left ankle, holding the towel with your hands over the right shoulder. Bend your knee about 90 degrees.

- Movement: Bend your left knee actively to full flexion without pulling on the towel/bed sheet. Lift your thigh off the floor by extending your hip to end range by contracting the left buttock. At this point, induce the stretch by pulling on the towel for three seconds. You should feel the stretch in the front of your thigh and in the groin. Release the pull and actively return your leg to the starting position. Repeat for the recommended repetitions on each side.

- WIIFM: Improves flexibility of the quadriceps at the front thigh and hip flexors within the groin. Isolated recruitment of the buttock for core stabilization.

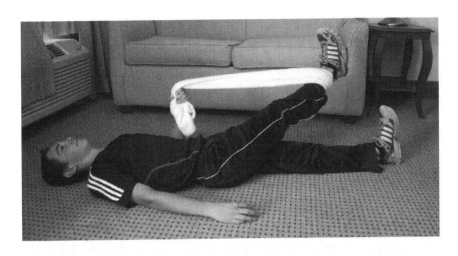

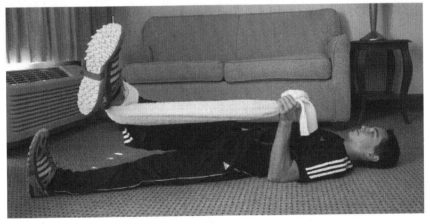

43. Iliotibial band stretch

- Starting Position: Lie on your back with both legs resting on the floor. Wrap a towel or a bed sheet—preferably longer to make the process easier—around the left ankle and arch of your foot. Hold across your body in your right hand.

- Movement: Actively lift your left leg up 2 to 3 feet off the floor keeping your knee straight. Move it across your body to the right keeping your toes pointing to the ceiling. At end range, pull out to the right with your right hand to induce the stretch down the outer thigh from the buttock to the hip and into the thigh. Hold for three seconds and return the leg actively to the starting position. Repeat for the recommended number of repetitions on each side.

- WIIFM: Improves flexibility of the lateral thigh, technically called the "iliotibial band."

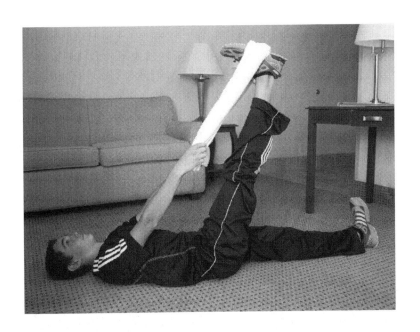

44. Hamstring stretch

- Starting Position: Wrap a towel or a bed sheet—
  preferably longer to make the process easier—around
  the arch of your left foot, holding at your chest with
  both hands. Lie on your back with both legs resting on
  the floor.

- Movement: Actively lift your left leg as far as you can,
  while keeping your knee straight and your foot flexed
  toward the knee. At end range, pull on the bed sheet to
  induce the stretch down the back of your thigh. Hold
  for three seconds and return the leg actively to the
  starting position. Repeat for the recommended number
  of repetitions on each side.

- WIIFM: Improves flexibility within the posterior
  thigh, called the "hamstrings," especially helpful after
  prolonged sitting.

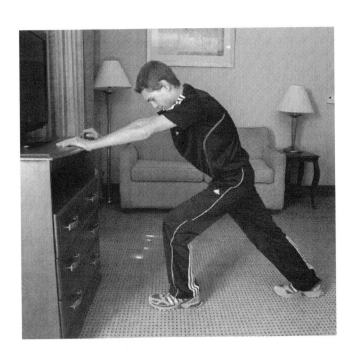

45. Standing calf stretch against wall

- Starting Position: Step your right leg forward while you continue to stand, facing the wall with your arms straight out at shoulder level and hands on the wall. Keep the left leg straight and back while the right leg remains bent at the knee, one step forward of the left. Point the toes of both feet toward the wall.

- Movement: Lean into the wall by bending your elbows and your right knee while keeping your left knee straight and both heels on the ground. Feel this stretch in the calf of the back leg. Complete the recommended number of repetitions on each leg, alternating sides.

- WIIFM: Improves calf flexibility, beneficial after prolonged sitting.

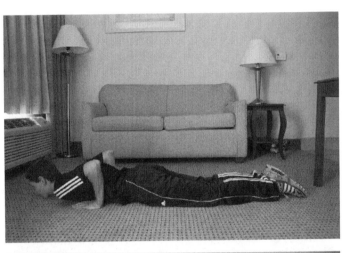

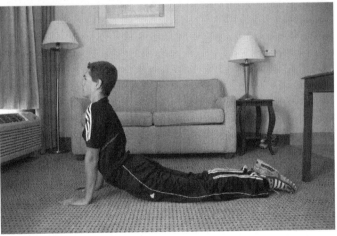

46. Press-up

- Starting Position: Lie on your belly with your hands under your shoulders in the push-up position.

- Movement: Relaxing your back, pressing up with your arms while keeping your pelvis sagging and in contact with the floor. Your arms should become the only places in your body where you feel muscles contracting.

- *Discontinue immediately if you already suffer from low back pain and this worsens the condition.*

- WIIFM: Reduces low back pain of disc origin and eases lumbar tightness due to prolonged flexed lumbar spine postures, such as slouching positions. Less aggressive exercise than press-up with a sag.

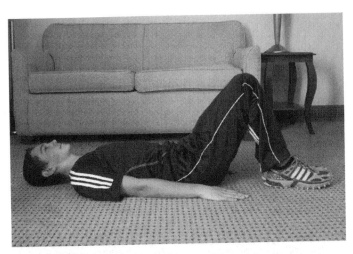

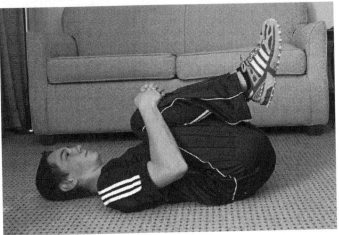

47. Double knee to chest

- Starting Position: With arms at your sides, lie on your back with your knees bent, feet together and flat on the floor.

- Movement: Actively raise both knees towards your chest while bending at the hips. Grab your knees with both hands and pull them to end range at your chest. Hold for the recommended time and return the legs to the starting position. Repeat for the recommended number of repetitions.

- WIIFM: Relieves low back stiffness by stretching the muscles and ligaments in that area. Beneficial after any prolonged sitting.

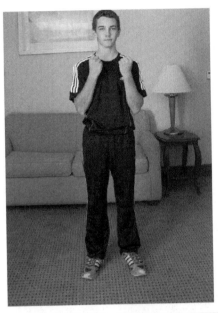

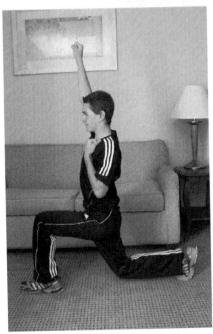
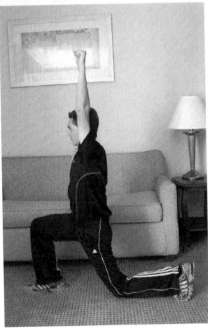

48. Static lunges with alternate overhead press

- Starting Position: Take a large step forward, with your elbows bent and fists clenched facing each shoulder. The distance from the toe of your back foot to the heel of your front foot should be longer than the distance from your knee to the ground when standing upright. Keep your torso erect and abdominal muscles tightened by pulling your belly button toward your spine and then under your ribs.

- Movement: Lower your body by flexing the front and rear knees, while keeping torso erect and abdominals tight throughout the motion. Your front knee should bend to no more than 90 degrees, never passing the mid-foot. Think of "sitting back and down" to help this process. You should feel your weight through the heel of your front foot, rather than the ball of your foot. While descending into the lunge, punch vertically upward with the arm opposite to the front leg. All along, make sure to turn your fist to face forward at maximal overhead reach. Push back up while lowering the arm to the starting position. Repeat with the other leg and arm, alternating sides until completing the recommended repetitions on each side.

- WIIFM: Improves balance and strength through controlled activation of hip, trunk and thigh musculature with a narrow base of support. Added overhead press challenges the body's ability to maintain balance, thereby enhancing core control and strengthening shoulder musculature. An advancement of the static lunge exercise.

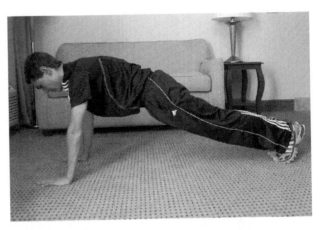

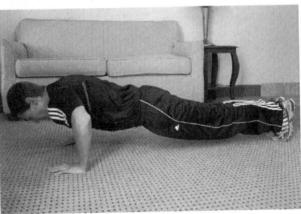

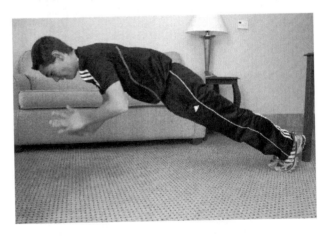

49. Push-up with clap

- Starting Position: With elbows straight, get in the push-up position with hands shoulder width apart and feet together. Keep your body in a straight line from ankles, through knees, hips, shoulders and ears.

- Movement: Lower your chest to the floor while maintaining your entire body in a straight line. Explode back up with arms lifting your hands of the floor, quickly clapping hands together and catching the descent again with your hands quickly returning to the floor. If unable to do this with your body fully straight from ankles to ears, rest on your knees instead of your toes. Alternatively complete this movement with your hands on the bathroom counter or furniture like an immovable desk or chest of drawers.

- WIIFM: Conditions core and strengthens chest and arm musculature. Advancement of push-up with added plyometric component of the clap.

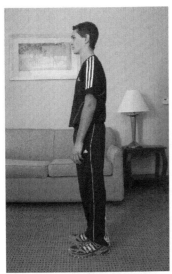
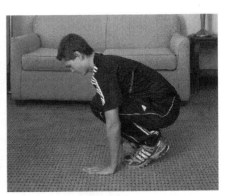
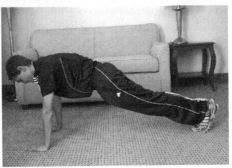
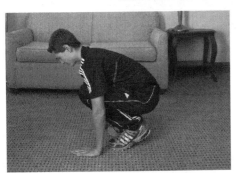
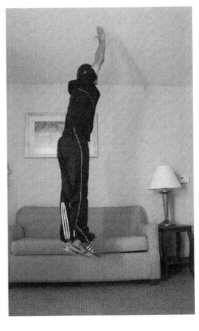

50. Burpees

- Starting Position: Stand with arms at your sides.

- Movement: With elbows straight, drop down into the full squat position with both hands on the floor just in front of your toes. Quickly kick your legs out backward so that you are at the top of a push-up position. Immediately return your legs to the squat position and jump as high as you can. As you land, repeat for the number of recommended repetitions.

- WIIFM: Develops core stability, leg strength and the anaerobic energy system—peaking the heart rate—through jump training or "plyometric," explosive maximal effort movements. Maintains aerobic condition of the elevated heart rate when combined with the other exercises of the routine.

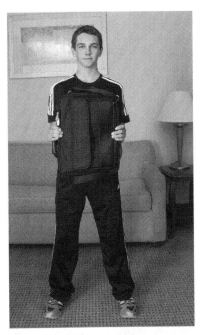

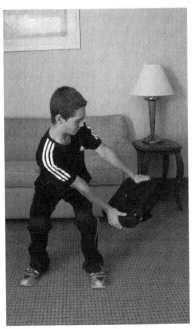

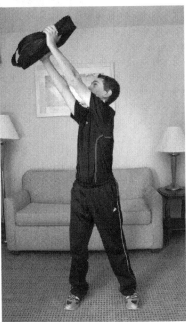

51. Squat with diagonal weight press

- Starting Position: With feet parallel to each other, stand with your feet a little wider than hip width apart, knees slightly bent. Hold a weighted object in front of you with both hands at waist level.

- Movement: While squatting back and down as if sitting in a chair, lower the weight toward the left outside ankle. Now, push forcefully up through your heels while raising the weight diagonally overhead to the right, your eyes following the weight. The mid position of the movement is fully extended in the legs. Do this while keeping the weight at maximal reach above your right shoulder, while turning your torso right as your head looks up in that direction. Return to the left squat position for one repetition. Complete the recommended repetitions. Repeat on the other side.

- WIIFM: Whole-body strengthening through multi-muscle recruitment that involves the arms, upper and lower back, core, hips and legs.

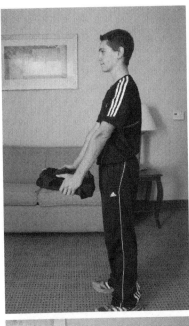

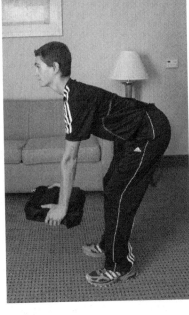

52. Straight leg deadlift

- Starting Position: Stand with your feet a little wider than hip width apart, knees slightly bent, feet parallel to each other and arms hanging in front of you, palms facing your thighs. You can hold a weight in both hands to increase exercise intensity.

- Movement: Flex forward at your hips while keeping your lower back neutral. To help this process, stick your buttocks out backward as you bend at the hips and keep your shoulders pulled back. Your arms will dangle straight down to the floor. When your torso is near parallel to the floor or you have reached maximum stretch of your hamstrings, extend your hips by contracting your buttocks—pushing through the front of your hips and return to the upright starting position. Repeat for the recommended repetitions.

- WIIFM: While avoiding unnecessary strain within the lumbar spine, this isolated hip hinge movement forces core control, strengthening the "paraspinal" regions against the spinal column, gluteus maximus and hamstring muscles.

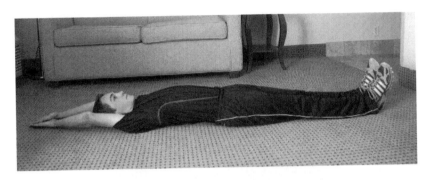

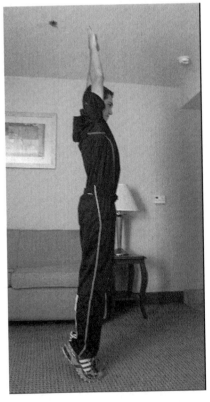

53. Back-to-toes-to-back-to-toes

- Starting Position: Lie on your back with your legs straight and arms overhead, palms up.

- Movement: Rapidly stand up onto your toes reaching your arms overhead, stretching as high as possible through your fingers. Immediately return to the starting position.

- WIIFM: Aerobic conditioning through rapid, repeated recruitment of large muscle groups in a complex movement.

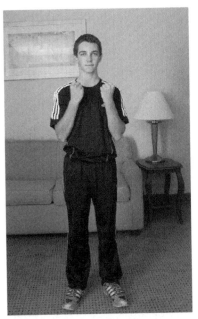

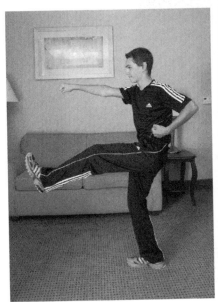
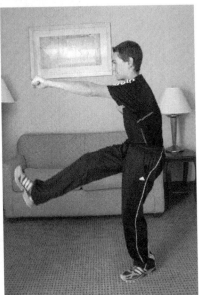

54. Alternate punch and kick

- Starting Position: Stand with feet comfortably apart and arms in flexed position with fists at chest level.

- Movement: Kick forward with your left leg and immediately return to the starting position. Punch out with the right fist at the same time. Return to starting position. Repeat kick and punch with the other side. Continue rapidly and with intensity for the recommended repetitions.

- WIIFM: Achieve dynamic balance through asymmetrical explosive movements requiring core stability and rapid muscle contractions. Stimulates aerobic energy systems when combined with the other exercises of the routine.

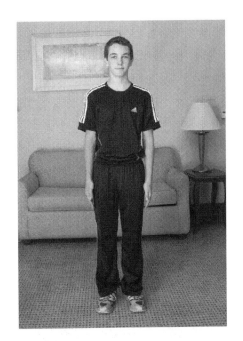

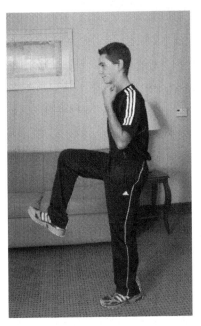 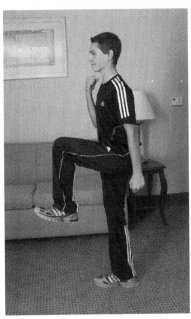

55. Marching with bicep curls

- Starting Position: Stand with feet together and arms at your side.

- Movement: Rapidly march on the spot, lifting your thighs parallel to the floor while bending your opposite elbow and bringing your fist to the front of your shoulder. Return to the starting position and repeat in quick succession with the other side. Continue for the recommended time.

- WIIFM: Develops dynamic balance through controlled marching, requiring hip stabilization while strengthening bicep muscles if a weight is used, or activating additional muscles to raise heart rate for aerobic conditioning without weights.

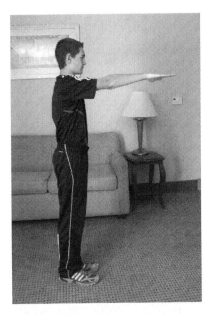

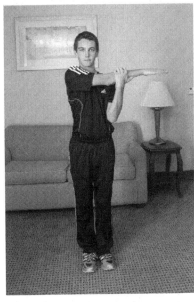

56. Posterior cuff stretch

- Starting Position: Stand with right arm in front of you at shoulder level, palm down.

- Movement: Actively move your right arm across your body toward the left shoulder. Push your elbow in toward the left shoulder with your left hand grasping the right elbow. You should feel a stretch in the back of the shoulder. If you feel a pinching sensation in the front of the shoulder you are impinging and should either pull lower down toward your left mid-chest or completely avoid this exercise. Hold for thirty seconds. Repeat for the recommended repetitions on each side.

- WIIFM: Improves flexibility of the posterior shoulder structures, an excellent preventative exercise for anterior shoulder pain.

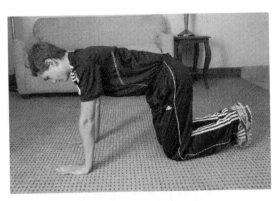

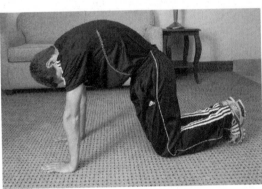

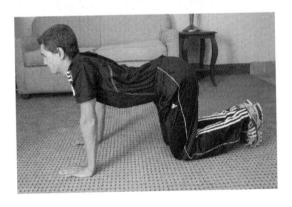

57. Cat-camel stretch

- Starting Position: Quadruped position on the floor or bed.

- Movement: Keep your elbows locked straight, arch your back up pushing through your arms—thereby rounding your shoulders. Meantime, tilt your pelvis posteriorly. Your spine arcs up toward the ceiling. Hold for two seconds. Now, sink down between your shoulders while letting your spine relax toward the floor and your pelvis tilt anteriorly. Hold for two seconds. Repeat for the recommended repetitions.

- WIIFM: Warm up of the core and spinal joints through gentle movement from extension in sunken position to flexion in the arched position.

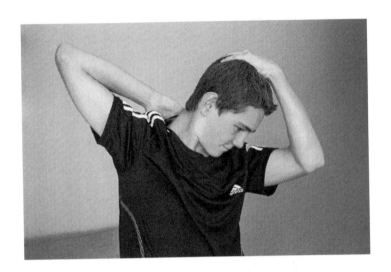

58. Levator scapulae stretch

- Starting Position: While seated, place your right hand behind your neck on the right shoulder blade with the elbow pointing to the ceiling. Turn your head halfway to the left and place your left hand on top of your head with your elbow in line with your forehead.

- Movement: Pull your head down with your left hand as if looking into the left pocket on your shirt, while keeping your right elbow vertical. Hold for thirty seconds. Repeat for the recommended repetitions on each side.

- WIIFM: Improves flexibility of the levator scapulae muscles at the back and side of the neck, particularly beneficial for headaches and neck stiffness due to cervical muscle tension. This muscle frequently has "the painful knot" just above the shoulder blade.

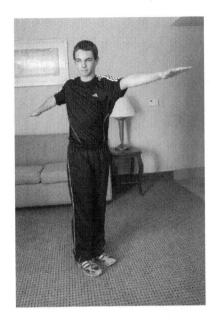

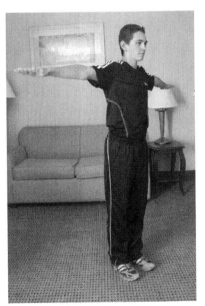
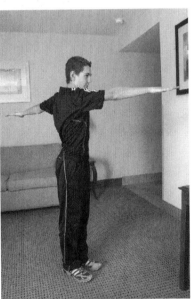

59. Standing trunk rotation, shoulder level arms

- Starting Position: Stand with feet hip width apart and arms out to your sides at shoulder level, palms down.

- Movement: Bracing your abdominal muscles by pulling your belly button in to your spine and up under your ribs, fully rotate your upper body to the left and then to the right, keeping your hips facing forward. Repeat each direction for the recommended repetitions.

- WIIFM: Separating the pelvis and legs, upper trunk rotation warms up the core muscles.

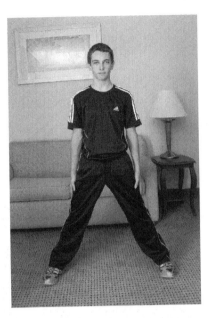

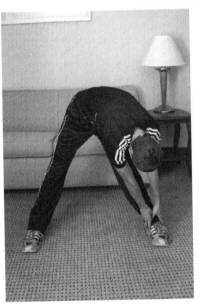
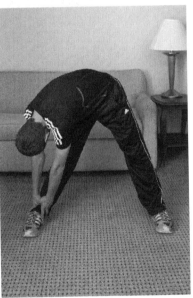

60. Flexion in standing wide stance (Giraffe stretch)

- Starting Position: Stand erect, arms at your side and with your feet wide apart, twice to three times your hip width.

- Movement: Bend forward diagonally, down the left leg toward the ankle. Start from the top by flexing your neck to look down while letting your arms dangle toward the floor, and then sequentially your shoulders, mid-back and low back. You should feel as if rolling down vertebrae-by-vertebrae from top to bottom. Reach with both hands as far as you can toward your ankle. Hold the stretch, felt in the back of your thighs and possibly in your low back—depending if you are tight there—for the recommended duration. Reverse the movement to return to the starting position. Keep your legs straight throughout the movement down and the return to the starting position. Repeat down the opposite leg. Alternate sides for the recommended repetitions.

- WIIFM: Achieve lumbar spine motion and hamstring flexibility through stretching the muscles and ligaments in your low back and hamstrings at the back of your thighs. Particularly beneficial after any prolonged sitting.

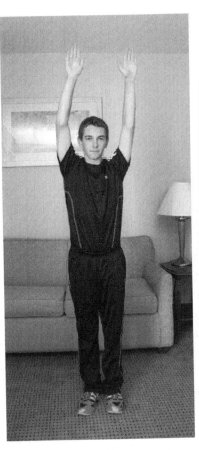
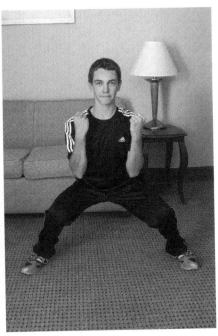

61. Side squat with overhead press

- Starting Position: Stand erect with feet hip width apart, arms extended fully overhead and palms facing forward. Tighten your abdominal muscles by pulling your belly button in toward your spine and up under your ribs.

- Movement: Take a large step to the right, feet parallel to each other and toes pointed forward. Sit back and down as if touching your buttocks to the seat of a chair in a controlled descent. Meantime, lower your arms by bending at the elbows and rotating your palms to face your shoulders at the bottom of the squat. Both knees flex until your thighs become parallel with the floor. You should feel weight through the heels, rather than the balls of your feet. Rise back to the starting position, pushing up and back to the left with your right leg. Forcefully reach high overhead, fully extending your arms and rotating your palms forward again. After doing the recommended repetitions to the right, repeat the movement to the left.

- WIIFM: Whole body strengthening through multi-muscle recruitment involving the arms, upper and lower back, core, hips and legs. Combining side squats with the overhead press emphasizes core strength.

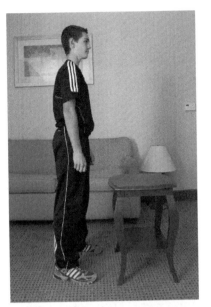

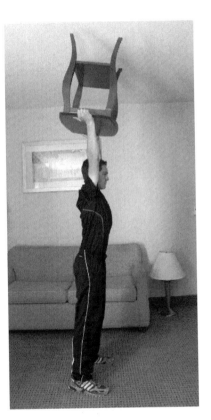

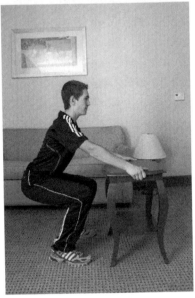

62. Chair overhead lift

- Starting Position: Stand behind a light wood chair, small table or other sturdy but small piece of furniture, arms at your sides and feet slightly wider than hip width apart.

- Movement: Squat back and down as though sitting in a chair. Your weight should be through the heels of your feet. Grab the upper portion of the back legs of the chair or small table. Now, push through the heels of your feet, going up to the standing position while simultaneously lifting the furniture overhead. Return to squat position and lower the furniture to the floor in a controlled manner. Repeat for the recommended repetitions.

- WIIFM: Whole body strengthening and core activation through multi-muscle recruitment involving the arms, upper and lower back, core, hips and legs.

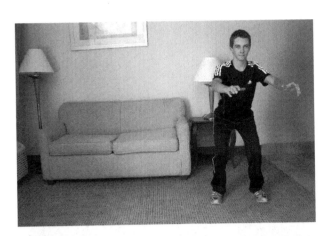

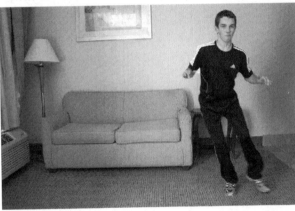

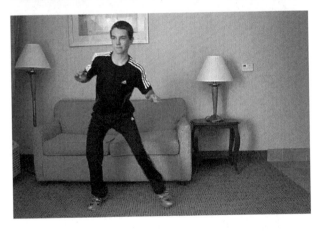

63. Side-to-side shuffle

- Starting Position: Clear the longest open floor space in the room. Stand sideways at one end of the space.

- Movement: Rapidly shuffle across the length of the room and back. Emphasize rapid, sideways foot movement and immediate direction changes at each end of the shuffle. Continue back and forth for the recommended time.

- WIIFM: Aerobic conditioning.

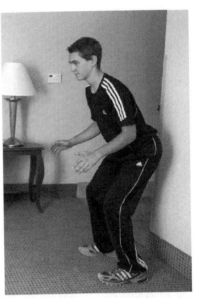

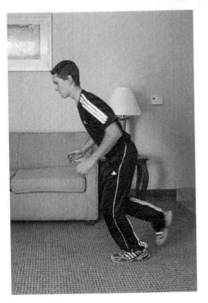

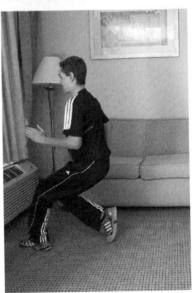

64. Forward-backward shuffle

- Starting Position: Clear the longest open floor space in the room. Stand at one end facing the open space.

- Movement: Rapidly run the length of the room and shuffle backward. Emphasize rapid, forward and backward movement with immediate direction changes at each end of the shuffle. Continue back and forth for the recommended time.

- WIIFM: Aerobic conditioning.

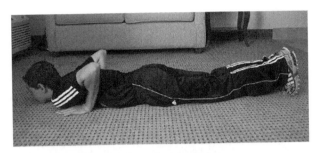

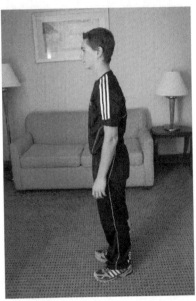

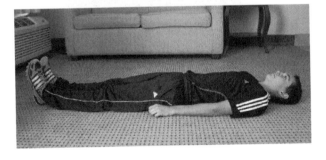

65. Stomach-to-back up and downs

- Starting Position: Lie on your belly with your hands under your shoulders in the push-up position.

- Movement: Rapidly stand erect and then immediately lower yourself to the floor again onto your back. Immediately, stand erect again and then lower yourself to the floor again into the starting position. Emphasize speed and standing fully erect. Repeat for the recommended time.

- WIIFM: Aerobic conditioning through rapid, repeated recruitment of large muscle groups in a complex movement.

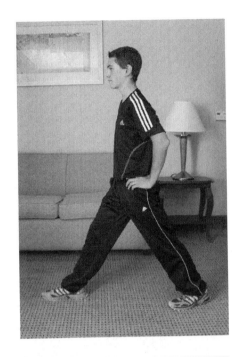

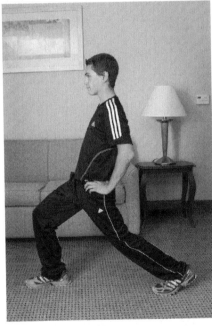

66. Standing hip flexor stretch

- Starting Position: Keeping hands on your hips, place the right foot out ahead of your body in a lunge position.

- Movement: Keeping your torso vertical, tighten your left buttock while pushing your left hip forward while shifting weight forward onto your right foot. Keep the left hip extended in this position. Feel a stretch in the left groin area. Repeat on the other side.

- WIIFM: Improves flexibility of hip flexors, especially beneficial after prolonged sitting.

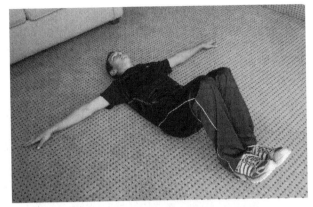

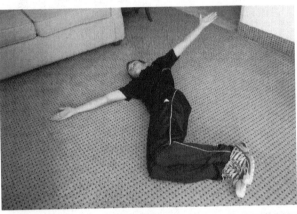

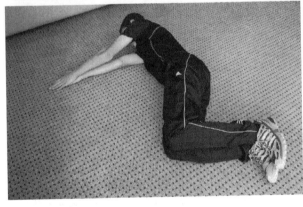

67. Hip crossover with trunk to follow

- Starting Position: Lie on your back on the floor with your knees bent about 90 degrees to 100 degrees. Keep your knees and feet together. Keep your heels on the ground and forefoot and toes pulled up toward your shins. Your arms point to the ceiling.

- Movement: Pull your belly button towards your spine and under your chest—making yourself skinny— thereby developing submaximal tension in your abdominal muscles. Rotate your legs to the left while keeping this tension. At end range, rotate your trunk to the left following your legs until lying on your left side. Reach forward through the fingers of your right hand thus bringing the scapular forward and feeling a stretch between the shoulder blades. Return the trunk to the starting position. Now, tighten the abdominal muscles again—making yourself skinny—and rotate your legs all the way to the right. At end range, rotate your trunk to the right following your legs until lying on your right side. Reach forward through the fingers of your left hand, thereby bringing the scapular forward and feeling a stretch between the shoulder blades. Return the trunk to the starting position. Continue until the recommended repetitions are completed on each side.

- WIIFM: Core warm up and recruitment. Promotes mobility of the lumbar spine, stretches the core muscles and ligaments and creates low-intensity activation of the abdominal muscles. Advancement from hip crossovers.

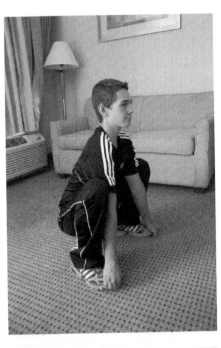

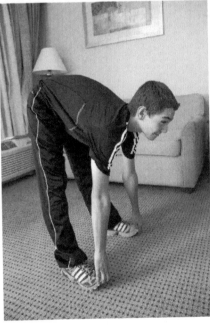

68. Sumo squat

- Starting Position: Stand with your feet wide enough that your buttocks can fit between your ankles. Squat down to grasp your toes with your hands, elbows inside your knees. Your weight should be through your heels, rather than the balls of your feet.

- Movement: Keep hold of your toes and straighten your legs as far as you can. You should feel stretching in the back of your thighs. Return to the starting position. Complete the recommended repetitions.

- WIIFM: Improves hamstring flexibility, hip mobility, core control and thoracic spine posture through scapular retraction.

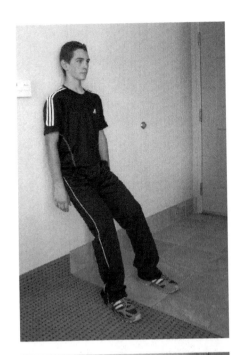

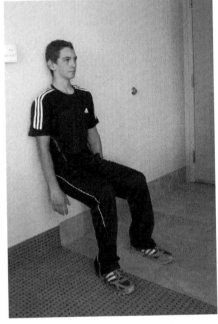

69. Wall squats feet flat

- Starting Position: Lean against the wall with your back, hands at your sides, and feet hip width apart.

- Movement: While walking—actually moving—your feet away from the wall, bend your knees and slide your back down the wall toward the floor. Descend into the squatting position until your thighs become parallel to the floor and knees are bent 90 degrees. Hold this position for the recommended duration, and then ascend back up to the starting position. Repeat for the recommended repetitions.

- WIIFM: Leg strengthening with core activation.

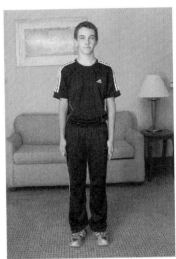

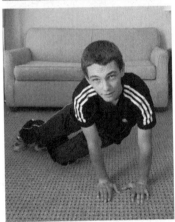

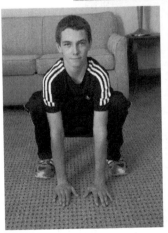

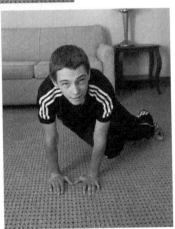

70. Half-burpee

- Starting Position: Stand with arms at your sides.

- Movement: Drop down into the full squat position with both hands on the floor just in front of your toes, elbows straight. Quickly kick your legs out to the right, elbows locked in extension. Immediately return your legs to the squat position with both hands on the floor in front of you and then stand up again. Repeat the movement with your legs going to the left. Continue for the number of recommended repetitions to each side, alternating directions.

- WIIFM: Intensive core activation and shoulder stability training.

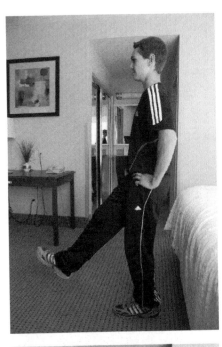

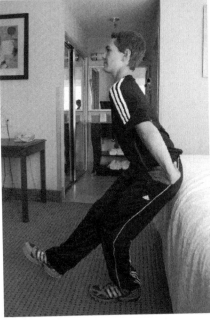

71. Butt-to-bed touch single leg squat

- Starting Position: Stand on one leg with your hands on your hips with the bed about a foot behind you.

- Movement: Lower your buttocks to touch the bed and return to the single leg stance position. Repeat for the recommended repetitions and then complete a set on the opposite leg.

- WIIFM: Progression from the regular squat to stimulate intensive core control through unilateral multi-muscle recruitment of the hips, legs and core.

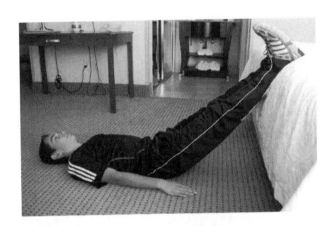

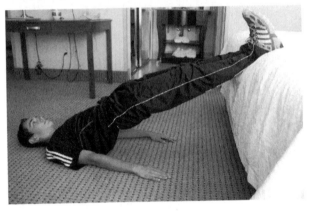

72. Heels-on-bed, straight-leg butt lift

- Starting Position: Lie on the floor on your back with your heels on the bed and legs straight.

- Movement: Brace your abdominals by pulling your belly button in to your spine and up under your ribs. Squeeze your buttocks together and push up through the front of your hips to lift your body off the floor. At the top of the movement you should have a straight line from your ankles to your knees, hips and shoulders. Your shoulders should rest on the floor, heels remaining on the bed. Hold this position for two to three seconds and return to the starting position. Repeat for the recommended number of repetitions.

- WIIFM: Hip extension benefiting the hamstrings and buttocks, and core recruitment for the paraspinals and abdominals.

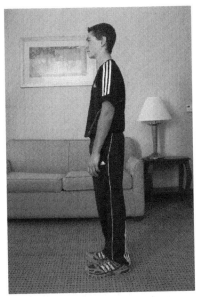
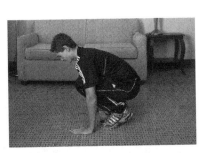
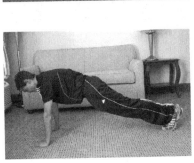
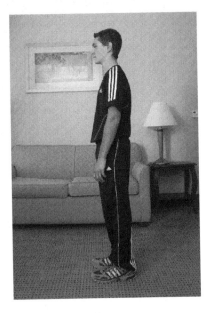

73. No-jump burpee

- Starting Position: Stand with arms at your sides.

- Movement: Drop down into the full squat position with both hands on the floor just in front of your toes, elbows straight. Quickly kick your legs out backward so that you are at the top of a push-up position. Immediately return your legs to the squat position and stand into an erect posture. Repeat for the number of recommended repetitions.

- WIIFM: Develops core stability, leg strength and the anaerobic energy system—peaking your heart rate—through plyometric, explosive maximal effort movements. Maintains elevated heart rate—aerobic conditioning—when combined with other exercises of the routine.

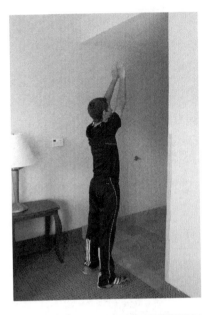

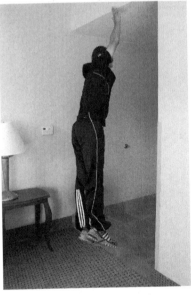

74. Overhead wall touch

- Starting Position: Stand facing a wall and raise both arms overhead reaching through your fingers as high as you can.

- Movement: Rapidly jump up and down on the balls of your feet, touching the wall with the tips of your fingers at the top of each jump. Always strive to achieve your goal of touching the wall as high and as many times as possible in the recommended time period.

- WIIFM: Develops rapid muscle recruitment around the ankles, improving proprioception, balance and hence ankle stability. Aerobic conditioning also results when combined with the other exercises within the routine.

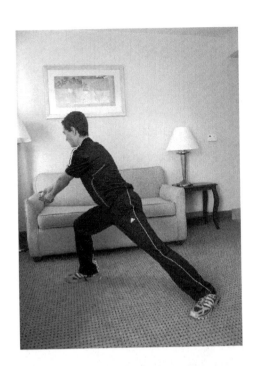

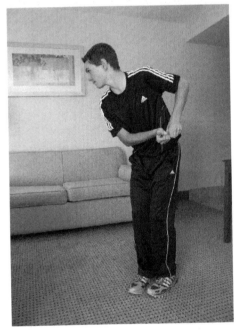

75. Left-to-right weight shift with rope pull

- Starting Position: Stand at one end of the room such that you can move to the right along a clear path.

- Movement: Lunge laterally with the right leg dropping your buttocks back and down while reaching out to the left with your arms, as if you were about to pull on a rope in a tug-of-war. Push up with your left leg to the standing position while making the rope-pulling movement with your arms, pulling to your chest. Continue back and forth across the room for the recommended repetitions on each side.

- WIIFM: Develops hip strength and control while activating the core in a slow, controlled movement.

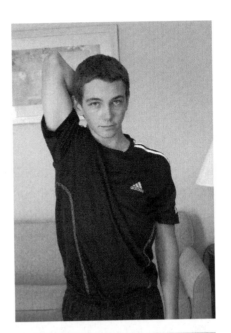

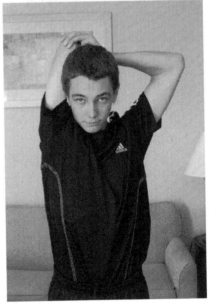

76. Tricep stretch

- Starting Position: Stand erect, place your right hand behind your neck so that your elbow points to the ceiling.

- Movement: With your left forearm behind your head, grab your right elbow with your left hand and pull behind your head to the left side. Keep your right elbow in a relaxed, flexed position. You should feel a stretch in the back of the upper arm.

- WIIFM: Improves flexibility of the triceps, at the back of the upper arm, and helpful for people suffering tension in the neck and shoulder area.

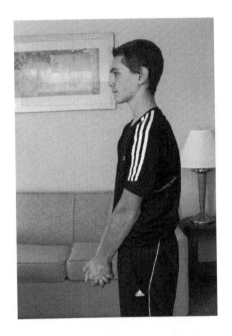

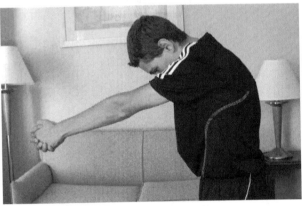

77. Standing upper thoracic stretch

- Starting Position: Stand with your fingers interlocked and your arms relaxed in front of you.

- Movement: While keeping your fingers interlocked and elbows straight, raise your arms to just below shoulder level. Reach out as far as you can in the plane of your arms by rounding your shoulders and pushing through your interlocked hands. Flex your neck at the same time, taking your chin to your chest. You should feel a stretch across the upper back. Hold for the recommended time.

- WIIFM: Relieves upper back and neck tension, sometimes caused by stress.

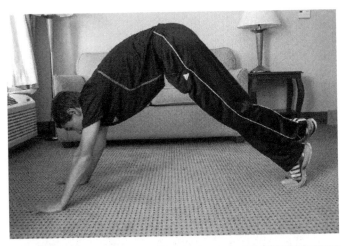

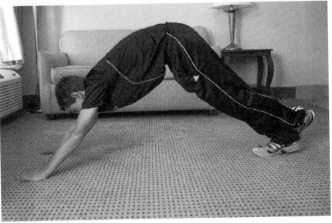

78. Prone gastroc-soleus stretch

- Starting Position: Get in the push-up position with arms straight and vertical beneath your shoulders. Cross the left ankle over the right Achilles just above the heel, keeping the right knee straight.

- Movement: Rise up on the toes of the right foot while keeping the right knee straight. Then, lower your heel toward the ground, knee still straight, and push the left heel down toward the floor with your left foot until feeling a stretch in the calf. Repeat for the recommended number of repetitions.

- WIIFM: Improves calf flexibility. Useful as a warm-up to prevent injury before progressing to more advanced strengthening exercises.

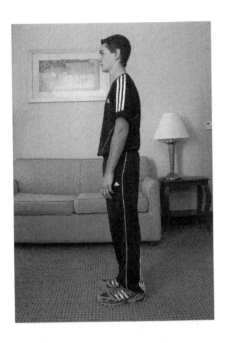 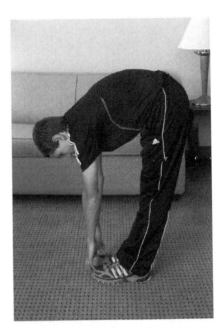

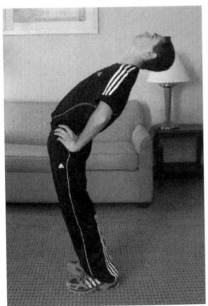 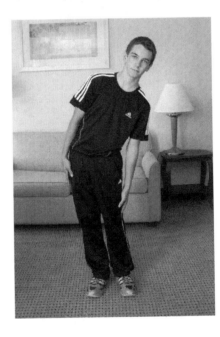

79. Flexion-extension-right-left side bending in standing

- Starting Position: Stand erect with your feet together and arms at your sides.

- Movement: Bend forward toward your toes. Start from the top by flexing your neck to look down, then sequentially your shoulders—while letting your arms dangle towards the floor—to your mid-back and then the low back. You should feel as if rolling down vertebrae-by-vertebrae from top to bottom. Reach toward the floor with both hands as far as you can. Reverse the movement to return to the starting position. Place your hands on your hips and bend backward, keeping your legs straight. Return to the starting position. Side bend to the right and then to the left. Repeat entire sequence for the recommended repetitions.

- WIIFM: Warm-up through end range, active movement of the lumbar spine in all directions.

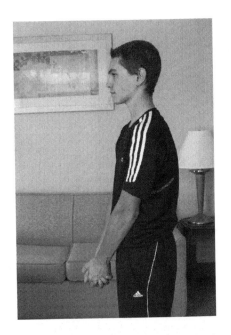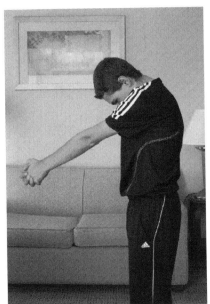
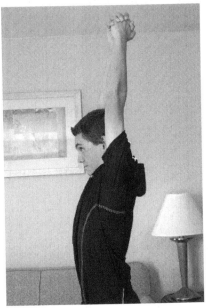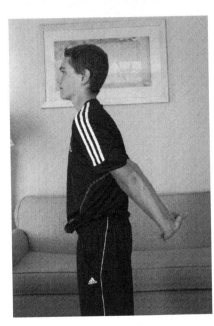

80. Upper thoracic to overhead to bicep stretch

- Starting Position: Stand with your fingers interlocked and your arms relaxed in front of you.

- Movement: Keeping your fingers interlocked and your elbows straight, raise your arms to just below shoulder level. Reach out as far as you can in the plane of your arms by rounding your shoulders and pushing through your interlocked hands. Meantime, flex your neck, taking your chin to your chest. Hold for five seconds. Slowly raise your arms overhead and reach maximally up to the ceiling. Again, hold for five seconds. Unlatch your fingers and reach with both arms behind you, again interlocking your fingers with elbows remaining straight. Keep your fingers linked, palms turned downward as far as possible. At the same time, raise your arms up behind you to feel a stretch in your bicep area on both sides. Hold for five seconds. Repeat the cycle for the recommended number of repetitions.

- WIIFM: Improves shoulder mobility in preparation for more advanced strengthening exercises or as a cool down, while also stretching the upper back and then the latissimus muscles and the biceps.

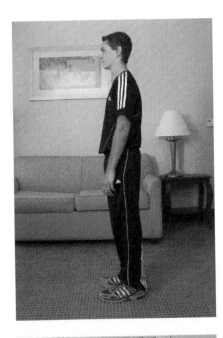

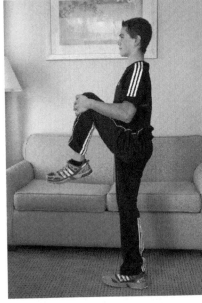

81. Knee-to-chest walk

- Starting Position: Stand with arms at your side with a clear pathway in front of you.

- Movement: Take a step forward with your right leg and bring your left knee towards your chest. Place your hands around your bent knee, which you then pull as far as possible toward your chest. Lower the left leg taking another step forward and pull your right knee into your chest with your hands around the bent knee. Continue stepping and stretching for the recommended repetitions.

- WIIFM: Develop hip, knee and ankle control for balance in single-leg stance while stretching the gluteus muscles.

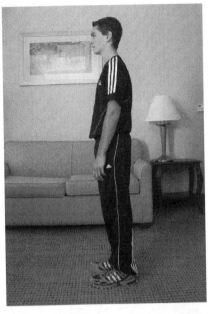

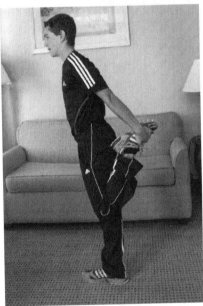
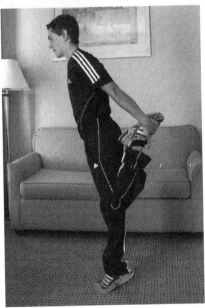

82. Walking quad stretch with heel raise

- Starting Position: Stand with arms at your side with a clear pathway in front of you.

- Movement: Take a step forward with your right leg and bring your left heel to your buttock. Grab around your left ankle with your left hand and pull the heel to your buttock, keeping your torso upright and your hip extended. You should feel a stretch in the front of your left thigh. Lower the left leg into another step forward, bend your right knee backward and pull your right heel to your right buttock as described above. Continue stepping and stretching for the recommended repetitions on each side.

- WIIFM: Develops hip, knee and ankle control for balance in single-leg stance. Stretches the quadriceps located at the front of the thigh.

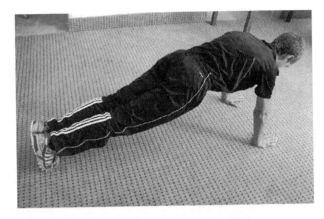

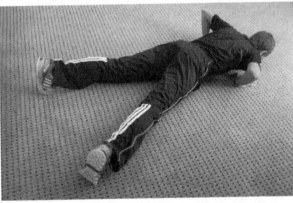

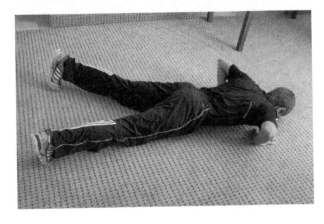

83. Push-up with hip abduction

- Starting Position: Get in the push-up position with hands shoulder width apart and feet together. With elbows straight, keep your body in a straight line from ankles, through knees, hips, shoulders and ears.

- Movement: Lower your chest to the floor maintaining your entire body in a straight line. Meantime, move your right leg out to the side as far as possible with the knee straight. As you push back up return your right leg to the starting position. Lower your chest to the floor again and now move your left leg out to the side as far as possible with the knee straight. As you push back up return your left leg to the starting position. Repeat for the recommended number of repetitions.

- WIIFM: Conditions core and strengthens chest and arm musculature. Advancement of push-up with added hip abduction.

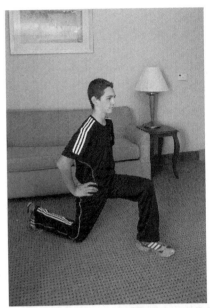

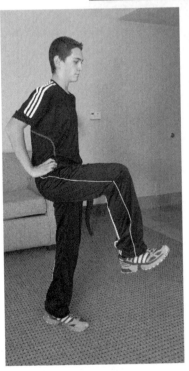

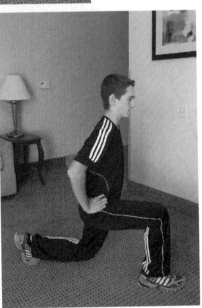

84. Reverse lunge to forward lunge

- Starting Position: With abdominals braced by pulling belly button toward your spine and under your ribs, stand erect with feet together and hands on your hips.

- Movement: Keeping your hands on your hips and torso erect, take a large step forward with your right leg. The distance from the toe of your back foot to the heel of your front foot should be larger than the distance from your knee to the ground when standing upright. Lower your body by flexing the front and rear knees. Your front knee should bend to no more than 90 degrees, never passing the mid-foot. To maximize results, think of "sitting back and down." You should feel your weight through the heel of your front foot rather than the ball. Now, push backward through the front leg, reverse the motion past the starting position and into a backward lunge. This time the other leg moves forward to become the front limb, bent a maximum 90 degrees. Continue stepping from a backward to a forward lunge for the recommended repetitions using the right leg and then switch to the left.

- WIIFM: Improves balance and strength through controlled activation of hip, trunk and thigh musculature with a narrow base of support.

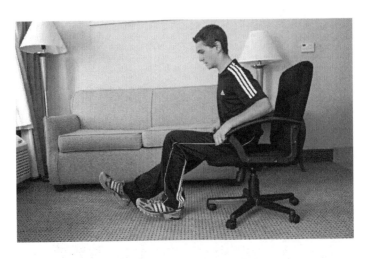

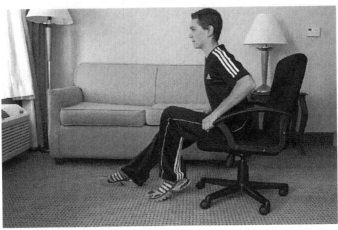

85. Stool scoot forward and backward

- Starting Position: Sit on a chair that has wheels, using your hands to hold on to the seat to prevent tipping during the exercise.

- Movement: With emphasis on speed of movement, pull yourself forward across the floor by digging your heels into the floor and forcefully bending your knees. Race across the room, then suddenly change direction, push backward across the floor to the starting position. Complete the recommended repetitions across the room for each set.

- WIIFM: Be dorky! Have fun! Pulling forward strengthens hamstrings and pushing backward strengthens quadriceps. Elevates heart rate when performed within a sequence targeted to stress the aerobic system.

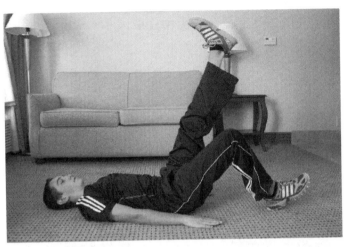

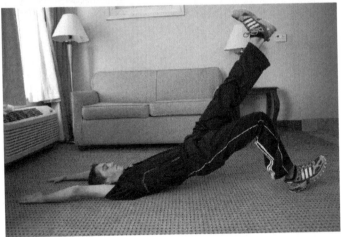

86. Single leg bridge with arm raise

- Starting Position: Lie on your back with your left knee bent 90 degrees, your foot on the floor in line with your left hip, ankle dorsiflexed – only the heel is on the floor. Hold your right leg straight toward to the ceiling. Hold this position throughout the movement. Keep arms palms down beside you on the floor.

- Movement: Tightening your abdominals by drawing your belly button in to your spine and up under your ribs and squeeze your buttocks together. Keeping these muscles contracted, lift your hips off the floor pushing up through the front of your left hip, reaching toward the ceiling with the heel of your right foot. Maintain a level pelvis. Meantime, raise both arms palms up above your head. You should feel your left buttock contract more than the right. Your trunk lifts up as a unit, both shoulders serving as your "fulcrum" of movement. You may not achieve full-hip extension, such as when both legs push up together during the regular gluteus bridge exercise. Hold the lifted position long enough to ensure that you have a maximal buttock contraction. Return to the starting position, while lowering your arms to your sides. Without releasing the gluteus contraction, touch the floor with your buttocks and lift buttocks and arms up again. Complete the recommended number of repetitions and then repeat on the other side.

- WIIFM: This asymmetrical task essentially "re-educates" the gluteus maximus and core musculature. Arm elevation improves thoracic spine mobility.

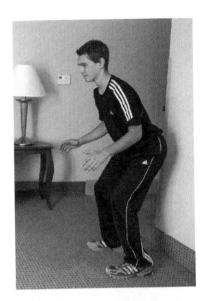

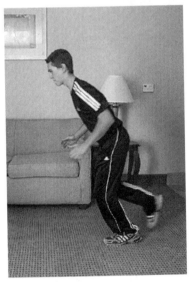

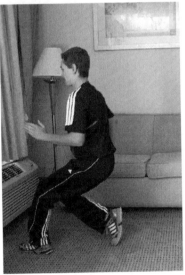

87. Forward shuttle room run

- Starting Position: Stand facing a 20- to 50-foot clear space.

- Movement: Run to the other side of the space as fast as possible, touch the floor with your left hand and run back to the starting point—where you also always touch the floor with your right hand. Repeat this shuttle run as fast as possible for the recommended duration.

- WIIFM: Aerobic conditioning.

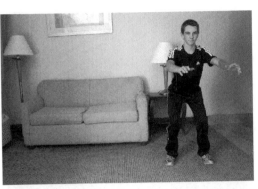

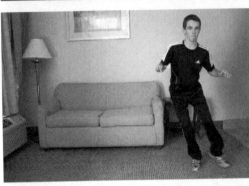

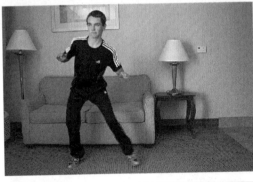

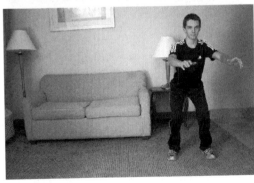

88. Lateral left-right room shuffle

- Starting Position: Stand sideways at one end of a 20- to 50-foot clear space, left side first.

- Movement: Shuffle to the left as fast as possible, touch the floor with your left hand at the end of the clearance and immediately shuffle back to the right—always touching the floor with your right hand at the starting point. Repeat this shuffle for the recommended duration as fast as possible.

- WIIFM: Aerobic conditioning.

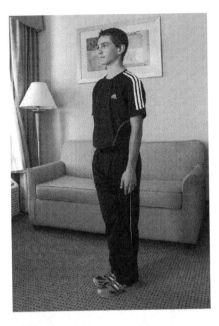

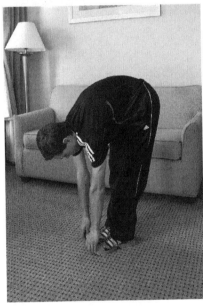

89. Standing crossed-leg hamstring stretch

- Starting Position: Arms at your sides while standing, cross the right leg in front of the left, keeping the left knee straight.

- Movement: Bend forward towards your toes. Start from the top by flexing your neck to look down, then—while letting your arms dangle toward the floor—sequentially your shoulders, followed by the mid-back and then the low back. You should feel as if rolling down vertebrae-by-vertebrae from top to bottom. Reach toward the floor with both hands as far as you can. You should feel a stretch down the back of your thighs, particularly the left. Hold for the recommended duration and return to the starting position. Repeat on the other side by placing the left leg over the right and then bending forward in the same way described above. Complete the recommended repetitions on each side.

- WIIFM: Improves lumbar and hamstring flexibility, while stretching the muscles and ligaments in your low back and hamstrings at the back of your thighs. Particularly beneficial after any prolonged sitting, such as after a lengthy flight or meeting.

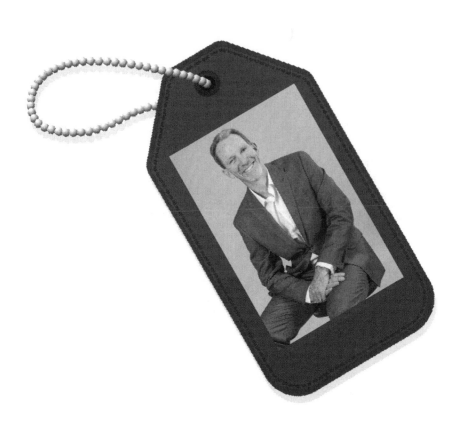

About The Author

André Meintjes, M.P.T., C.F.E., Ph.D., was forced by personal circumstances to make a drastic and life-saving lifestyle change after discovering a 95-percent blockage of the major coronary artery to his heart while running in 2003. He successfully completed this urgent transition by following simple principles and avoiding complicated processes so frequently publicized. He avoids medications and maintains his vibrant health through smart, simple methods of eating and exercising.

Doctor Meintjes has traveled extensively worldwide, and has experienced firsthand the challenges that being away from home can impose on efforts to maintain healthy living. Following more than a decade of clinical work, he originated and developed the concept of this book, utilizing his personal experience and his extensive post-professional education. A Certified Functional Evaluator, Doctor Meintjes has earned a Ph.D. in physiology and a Master's Degree in Physical Therapy.

The Doctor has practiced as a physical therapist since 1997. In 2002, he opened an outpatient physical therapy private practice, Custom Physical Therapy, which has grown into a thriving business with three locations and 20 employees, all in the Reno-Sparks area of Nevada.

Throughout life Doctor Meintjes has participated in various sports ranging from tennis, squash, cricket, hockey and racquetball, to racing road and mountain bikes, and rowing for his university. He presently rides his mountain bike, passionately enjoying the beautiful Sierra Nevada around Lake Tahoe and Reno with his wife, Coral, and their two teenage sons, Ian and Tate. Coral patiently and lovingly puts up with the family's three adrenaline-junkie "boys." The Doctor refrains from being picky about mountain bike trails: "Just show me some single track!"

CONTACT INFORMATION

Contact me and let me know how you are doing with this program. I would love to hear from you.

Have fun!

André

André Meintjes, M.P.T., C.F.E., Ph.D.
takechargehealthspeaker@gmail.com
20MinuteTravelWorkout.com
Facebook.com/ImpiloHealth